T0213767

Rethinking the Aging Transition

Kallol Kumar Bhattacharyya

Rethinking the Aging Transition

Psychological, Health, and Social Principles
to Guide Aging Well

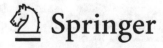

Kallol Kumar Bhattacharyya (iD)
School of Aging Studies
University of South Florida
Tampa, FL, USA

ISBN 978-3-030-88872-5   ISBN 978-3-030-88870-1   (eBook)
https://doi.org/10.1007/978-3-030-88870-1

This Springer imprint is published by the registered company Springer Nature Switzerland AG
The registered company address is: Gewerbestrasse 11, 6330 Cham, Switzerland

This work and accomplishment are dedicated to my adored God, late Sri Sri Manimohan Goswami.

Foreword

This book covers a lot of ground in gerontology. It is an evidence-based treatise covering many important age-related topics such as retirement, healthy aging, caregiving, mental health, dementia, diversity, longevity, technology, thanatology, and spirituality. However, the unique aspect of this volume relates to the author's personal reflections on how these topics are differentially addressed in Eastern and Western cultures. Dr. Kallol Kumar Bhattacharyya is an Indian-trained physician and American-educated gerontologist, and his views reflect the ideas of one who has been able to select the best of both disciplines and cultures to provide guidance on some of the most important issues facing the aging of the world population. As his mentor in the doctoral program in aging studies, I can attest that he has clearly gone beyond what can be taught in one program. His integration of Eastern and Western thought and his promotion of the time-honored practices of yoga and meditation are very much in tune with the accumulating empirical research in support of these practices. Dr. Bhattacharyya displays a true biopsychosocial approach that deftly merges science with person-centered care. I expect all readers will gain new perspectives on familiar aging transitions common to all cultures.

Victor Molinari
Professor, School of Aging Studies
University of South Florida
Tampa, FL, USA

Preface

I started my professional journey as a primary care physician almost two decades ago. As a clinician, a substantial amount of my time was spent educating my patients about taking care of their health in a holistic way. Different age levels, even different cognitive statuses of patients, made this job more challenging. After many years of practice as a self-employed practitioner, as well as practice in different government and private institutions, I found my work did not yield any innovative thoughts regarding managing patients; instead, it was gradually becoming a monotonous one for me. I wanted to have the education needed to reach beyond medical model treatments and provide my patients, particularly older adults, with more holistic management that maximizes their quality of life. This may be achieved through person-centered care that includes medical care but focuses on the quality of life and wellbeing.

I wanted to return to the academics from that passion for achieving what I wanted to pursue in my future. In professional practice, the majority of my patients were older adults suffering from various chronic diseases, and I really felt for them. Therefore, my stepping into Gerontology was not a surprise, at least for me. My goal has been to establish an identity as an academic researcher and a change agent who can conduct interdisciplinary scholarship with clinical expertise. I believe that the advanced study in Gerontology has enhanced my significant clinical education and experience and prepared me for this role. This combination of skills allows me to contribute meaningfully to improve the quality of care and the quality of life of older adults, particularly those living with debilitating chronic conditions, such as dementia. However, the step of studying abroad was a huge gamble for me, particularly after a long gap from academics, though I took that leap as a non-traditional student.

In this book, I incorporated the gradual changing pattern in the interdisciplinary aging processes, from the perspective of a physician as well as a social scientist, and tried to compare and contrast the two cultures. I believe the theme of this book about how to promote oneself as a change agent in the aging world would impress every reader rethinking the aging process of an individual. I believe this book has a strong academic value from a multicultural perspective and is helpful for Gerontology

graduate and undergraduate students; however, the main aim of this book is awareness generation. Therefore, this would be an important resource for a diverse group
of populations globally, such as clinical and non-clinical caregivers, even for elementary school teachers who teach our basic moral education, and of course, for
policymakers. Also, as a textbook, specialized courses in psychology, public health,
social work, theology, and diversity might use it. Therefore, I hope this book will be
beneficial for a wide group of readers.

Tampa, FL, USA   Kallol Kumar Bhattacharyya

Acknowledgments

I want to thank my former professors Drs. Jennifer Craft Morgan, Elisabeth Burgess, and Wendy Simonds for their input and guidance. I am also thankful to Drs. Ross Andel, Gizem Hueluer, Lindsay Peterson, and John Bowblis for their constructive criticism during my progress. I am particularly thankful to the late Dr. Kathryn Hyer, who provided me with the much-needed support; I am grateful for the direction I received from her. I want to thank Dr. Victor Molinari for being a patient and encouraging advisor throughout my journey as a doctoral student. His inputs were also a great asset for this book. I would also like to thank all the friends, colleagues, and professors with whom I was able to work during my journey to achieve my goals.

I am thankful to Ms. Janet Kim, Senior Editor at Springer Nature, and the entire publishing team for their patient cooperation throughout the process of publication. I am grateful to my parents, the late Mr. Kalyan Kumar Bhattacharyya and Mrs. Gita Bhattacharyya, and my grandparents for their continuous blessings. I am thankful to my sister Mrs. Kakali Bhattacharyya and my in-laws, Mr. Santanu Bhattacharya and Mrs. Papiya Bhattacharya, for their continuous encouragement. I would not have been able to complete this book without their love and support.

Finally, my wife Paramita Bhattacharya and my son Shailpik are the main strength and the constant source of support for me. I was amazed by how Paramita did the initial editing of several chapters of this manuscript and consistently was patient with me. This book may be an official achievement for me, but unofficially, all credit goes to them.

Last but not the least, I want to express my heartiest gratitude to all those individuals with or without disorders (earlier, I used to call them "my patients") who came to me for clinical suggestions on different occasions. Without their blessings, it would not have been possible for me to come to the point where I am today.

Contents

List of Figures

About the Author

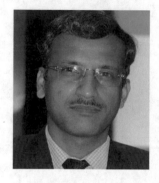

Kallol Kumar Bhattacharyya, MBBS, MA, PhD (Candidate), is a physician gerontologist with a general interest in providing older adults with more holistic health care that maximizes their quality of life. He worked as a family physician in India for nearly two decades. As a mid-life career changer, he completed his master's degree in Gerontology from Georgia State University, USA. Dr. Bhattacharyya is currently researching dementia at the School of Aging Studies, University of South Florida (Tampa), USA, where he is a doctoral candidate and undergraduate instructor. He expects to complete his PhD in Spring 2022. His research interests include mindfulness activities to improve the quality of life of persons with dementia, improvement of health policy for older adults, longevity, and healthy aging. Dr. Bhattacharyya is particularly focused on some alternative therapeutic interventions for Alzheimer's disease and related dementia. He is also working on the individualized care provided in institutional settings, especially nursing homes, and is interested in investigating how residents' satisfaction levels and subsequent complaints (if any) help identify flaws in the care delivery system.

Chapter 1
Introduction

The airplane has completed its final turn on the runway track. Now it is ready to run. A feeling of a light jerk, within a moment, it started running, faster and faster, and within a few seconds, it detached itself from the ground. Glowing lights are becoming smaller and smaller. The airplane is climbing higher and higher, saying goodbye to midnight's sleeping Kolkata. There is a transition of base underfoot, from land to air. Is it? Underfoot is the same floor mat, which was there a few minutes ago, when the plane was standing at the airport; still, there is a sensation of floating, a feeling of a journey through the dark sky, toward the darker one, hoping for a brightening light.

The same was the feeling of at least one of the passengers inside the plane. A transition of life from a clinician to a gerontologist, leaving an established career, a journey toward an extreme uncertainty. The last couple of months were very hectic, with a feeling of adventure in every step. However, time passed with busy arrangements for a dream. When the plane was standing at the airport, it was a feeling of reviewing the decision …was it right? When the plane started running, it was a feeling of helplessness …now I cannot stop this journey …we are leaving, at last, leaving everything behind. And now in the air, it is a feeling of anxiety …anxiety for a new environment, anxiety for a new life, anxiety for new resources. A feeling of helplessness that I will no longer be a practitioner there. An uneasiness for adjustment, from a professional's life to a nontraditional student's life. A discomfort, thinking about how I will look like in this new personality in the eyes of my closest two life companions. New lifestyle, new friends, new habitat, compromise, comments, criticism, everything just compelled me enough to close my eyes, with a sensation of floating in the air.

© The Author(s), under exclusive license to Springer Nature Switzerland AG 2021
K. K. Bhattacharyya, *Rethinking the Aging Transition*,
https://doi.org/10.1007/978-3-030-88870-1_1

1.1 Gerontology: The Option

Hippocrates wrote, "Wherever the art of medicine is loved, there is also a love of humanity" (Bertuzzi et al., 2020, p.61). I have chosen gerontology because I also believe in this strong interrelation between medicine and humanity. I worked as a family physician in Kolkata (India) for nearly two decades. In my professional life, I found that the majority of my patients were older adults and suffered from different chronic diseases. These patients were practically a burden to their family members in our present socioeconomic structure, where they found themselves neglected and helpless. I had a close dealing with these people, and I felt for them.

Modern medical advancements have increased longevity across the globe. Although the increased longevity is considered a public health victory (Bhattacharyya et al., 2021), it has some serious concerns, too, because of its growing demand for medical and social care. On many occasions, the growth of the older adult population is emerging as a socioeconomic concern that is increasing day by day. Many older adults are in critical need of better support for healthy aging or aging well, but there are only a few professionals in the field of gerontology, at least in my country India. Often people become confused by the terms gerontology and geriatrics. While gerontology is the complete study, i.e., social, cultural, psychological, cognitive, and biological aspects, of aging, Geriatrics is a branch of medicine that deals with the healthcare of older adults. Ideally, geriatrics is a part of interdisciplinary gerontology, which is a relatively new but rapidly growing domain in the field of caregiving. This growth is prevalent not only in India but also globally. As a clinician, I was serving the poor in India with dedication. A substantial amount of my time was spent educating my patients about taking care of their health. Different age levels, even different cognitive statuses of patients, made this job more challenging. However, coming toward the midpoint of my professional life, I realized that I could make more significant changes in society by generating insights about healthy aging as a researcher in addition to providing health education as a clinician. To be honest, I felt a deep need for new challenges. I decided to get the education needed to reach beyond medical model treatments and provide older adults with more holistic management that maximizes their quality of life while living with different chronic disorders (especially dementia). This better management can be achieved through person-centered care that includes medical care and focuses on quality of life and well-being. Therefore, I decided to jump into this field, not just to build a career but also from passion.

Another and probably the most powerful impact influencing my trajectory was that my grandmother suffered from Alzheimer's disease, and my mother was showing the early clinical manifestations of that disorder. I witnessed the disease process, not only as a clinician but also as a family member and care partner. Therefore, my experience in handling these situations was better than many others who experienced these problems. The death of my grandmother was a significant loss for me, as I had a strong bond with her and still feel a strong childhood nostalgia from my life with her. Today, the United States is in the midst of developing strong coalitions and revolutionizing the management of aging and dementia. This context has also influenced my thinking.

1.2   Tying Disparate Themes Together

The transition phase of pre-older adult to older adult controls the well-being of the concerned person remarkably economically, physically, and psychologically. All these issues have a profound influence on the morbidity and life span of the individual in later life. There is a dearth of literature covering various challenges faced by older adults from a global perspective. This discussion highlights some of the unique psychological, health, and social challenges faced by older adults globally and issues like positive psychology, spirituality, and longevity in the context of increasing numbers of older adults in every part of the globe. This narration also delineates some optimistic hopes from the ancient Indian philosophical thoughts of lifestyle. This discussion is a kind of phenomenology, views on the lifestyles of older adults in the two most popular democracies, and a comparative study based on the review of a few evidence-based pieces of literature on gerontology. This is a description of transition, issues toward healthy aging, caregiving, and an attempt to generate awareness among the general population to provide older adults a better quality of life. This book seeks to build an understanding of the fundamental relation of aging with various health and socioeconomic factors, such as physicians, retirement, caregiving, disease processes, social relations, diversity, longevity, technology, death, and spirituality. Finally, drawing ideas from a variety of resources, including books on multicultural aging, theories of aging, healthy aging, and dementia, and incorporating various arguments and both qualitative and quantitative data, this book targets each reader to be a change agent and a bridge in a smooth transition in the world of caregiving. This knowledge of the landscape of activities would help us rectify and improve strategies for supporting people living with different chronic disorders, including dementia, at a deeper, more meaningful level.

In the relatively short history of the social sciences and its branch that deals with aging studies, theory building is gradually becoming an increasing trend and an important aspect to establish a conceptual model (Alley et al., 2010; Bengtson et al., 1997). Although there is still no consensus on how to build an all-encompassing theory of aging, multiple theories currently represent several domains of the aging process to understand and explain aging phenomena systematically. Without following a theory, either explicitly or implicitly, the process of structuring and interpreting how and why aging (and various other processes) occurs often remains obscure; also, replicating the information gathered from the study remains obscure. The importance of theories is often trivialized. However, suppose the explanation in a study is not backed by theoretical assumptions, which were evident by research; in that case, it is difficult to justify whether the methodological approaches and the results are grounded to support assumptions. Scholars often consider theories as to the linkage between the theoretical knowledge of the researcher and its applied aspect (Hendricks et al., 2010). Therefore, in the following chapters, various theories related to aging processes would be the central aspect to advance the discussion on different aspects of aging. Various theoretical formulations, such as person centered, Hinduism, biopsychosocial, and positive psychology, have guided the discussions to address the subject matter in different chapters and the manuscript as a whole. The late middle age and early old age transitional period and East-West comparisons would reflect a unique perspective of this book, elaborating why rethinking is essential regarding a successful transition to the aging world. The following chapters attempt to tie various disparate themes together, focusing on the period of transition between late middle age and early old age (discussed in Chap. 3 on aging and retirement), emphasizing analysis of the differences between Eastern and Western cultures (the central aspect in aging and caregiving (Chap. 5), aging and diversity (Chap. 8), and aging and spirituality (Chap. 12)), and promoting a person-centered holistic biopsychosocial approach to aging that maximizes their quality of life while living with different chronic disorders (the key element in aging and physicians (Chap. 2), aging and mental health (Chap. 6), aging and dementia (Chap. 7), and aging and longevity (Chap. 9)).

References

Alley, D. E., Putney, N. M., Rice, M., & Bengtson, V. L. (2010). The increasing use of theory in social gerontology: 1990-2004. *The Journals of Gerontology. Series B, Psychological Sciences and Social Sciences, 65*(5), 583–590. https://doi.org/10.1093/geronb/gbq053

Bengtson, V. L., Burgess, E. O., & Parrott, T. M. (1997). Theory, explanation, and a third generation of theoretical development in social gerontology. *The journals of gerontology. Series B, Psychological Sciences and Social Sciences, 52*(2), S72–S88. https://doi.org/10.1093/geronb/52b.2.s72

Bertuzzi, A. F., Gennaro, N., Marrari, A., & Santoro, A. (2020). The blurred line between the art and science of medicine. *Radiotherapy and Oncology, 150*, 61. https://doi.org/10.1016/j.radonc.2020.05.030

Bhattacharyya, K. K., Molinari, V., & Hyer, K. (2021). Self-reported satisfaction of older adult residents in nursing homes: Development of a conceptual framework. *The gerontologist*, gnab061. Advance online publication. https://doi.org/10.1093/geront/gnab061

Hendricks, J., Applebaum, R., & Kunkel, S. (2010). A world apart? Bridging the gap between theory and applied social gerontology. *The Gerontologist, 50*(3), 284–293. https://doi.org/10.1093/geront/gnp167

Chapter 2
Aging and Physicians

2.1 Bioethics and Aging

Regarding the biopsychosocial model of disease management, physicians always considered a dualistic approach. It was probably Plato, who first realized that although there are distinct groups of physicians for the body and the soul, their roles cannot be independent (Drossman & Ruddy, 2021). In this context, ethics and morality play vital roles in all branches of medical science; while the word morality indicates a personal characteristic, the word ethics is used in the professional arena. As patient management is broadening its interdisciplinary nature, the significance of ethical principles is gradually increasing. The term "bioethics" is a subdivision of "ethics," and "bioethics and aging" is a subfield of "bioethics." Bioethics is considered a sort of guideline for all medical professionals to follow (McCullough, 2000). The purpose of ethics is somewhat similar to that of education, which indicates what is acceptable or unacceptable and what should and should not be done. Many principles of medical ethics have been used for centuries. For instance, during the fourth century BCE, Hippocrates, the great physician-philosopher, guided physicians to help people without doing any harm (Pappas et al., 2008). Likewise, showing respect for persons and offering justice have been present in societies from the earliest times. The Belmont report suggested three basic principles that we should follow while performing research involving human subjects: respect for persons, beneficence, and justice (Sims, 2010). These principles should be the guidelines not only in the research arena but also for every caregiver.

In medical practice, the major ethical principles that are expected to be maintained are autonomy, beneficence (doing the best for the patients), non-maleficence (not to harm), and justice (Raus et al., 2018). In healthcare, autonomy is considered as the right of competent adults to take informed decisions about their medical care. The principle guides the requirement to seek the consent or informed agreement of the patient before proceeding with any investigation or treatment. However, for all practical purposes, is this maintained in every step? Growing complexities in health-care networks involve more commercial activities; perhaps the quality of healthcare is improving, but the quality of maintaining ethics still remains questionable. In the current scenario of medical practice, two areas need considerable attention. McCullough (2000) highlighted the first one as end-of-life decision-making, where the healthcare professional is not the authority; instead, the patient should be in authority. There are some moral responsibilities of physicians caring for elderly patients; it is argued that these responsibilities are not rationalized simply in the patient's best interests from the physician's understanding. Instead, they should be considered based on the patient's past autonomy, that is, the values and beliefs that the patient held prior to the loss of competence. Family members have a key role to play in assisting the physician in constructing this "value history." The advance directives play a crucial role both in terminal illnesses and loss of decision-making capacity. Another questionable sector is physician-assisted suicide. The US Supreme Court has ruled that while there is no constitutionally protected right to physician-assisted suicide, there is also no constitutional bar to it (McCullough, 2000). Whereas in India, passive euthanasia has recently become legalized under certain mandatory guidelines (Das, 2019).

The second domain highlighted by McCullough is long-term care decision-making (McCullough, 2000). In contemporary American society, this is a difficult situation for many informal caregivers, especially women. However, it seems the problem prevails not only in the United States; instead, this is also a global problem. Various complex issues are arising day by day in the sectors of both caregiving at home and institutional caregiving. What should be the role of caregivers when the patients lack decision-making capacity? Due to the invasion of businessmen, now the medical profession is not considered "noble," at least the way Hippocrates thought. In this contemporary world of business, how far is the word bioethics sig-nificant? Are we maintaining the confidentiality of treatment? Variation in countries exists only in the perspectives, but the main point remains the same. The utilitarian approach suggests going for the consequences of a choice that promote the best result. In contrast, the deontological approach argues for the actions to respect invi-olable human rights, irrespective of their consequences (Mandal et al., 2016). We are in an ethical dilemma in the perspectives of demarcation between the utilitarian and the deontological approaches of ethical theories. We are in a conundrum of which side we should choose. Alternatively, whether, at all, do we have any options to choose any side. Medicalization has crucified the most honest caregivers. We are only part of the system and cannot do anything from within. Somehow morality is overshadowed by the "new" ethics. Honesty, integrity, respect, compassion, cour-age, self-sacrifice, and self-interest, all these terms are apparently melodious and have some differences in different cultural perspectives. However, globalization has made everything a hotchpotch. Some scholars consider that healthcare profession-als are aggressive with treatment in the United States, which is reflective of a culture that, to a certain extent, wants to deny infirmity and death by overtreating it. On the other hand, not giving any treatment at all may reflect a similar ageistic bias. However, it is crucial to learn that how we as clinicians fall on this "philosophical" continuum would hopefully keep us from confusing our worldview with that of our patients and allow our patients to take their own decisions based on their own values.

Regarding maintaining uniformity in social justice, the egalitarian approach suggests that individuals should receive healthcare in equal proportion to their health needs (McCullough, 2000). In contrast, the libertarian approach suggests that individuals should receive healthcare benefits in proportion to the amount they paid for it (McCullough, 2000). Who will decide whether someone should be treated based on the libertarian or egalitarian approach of healthcare? Is there any role of an individual in the systems, even in so-called democracies? Is there any country that exists in the world where democracy or a republic state is still maintained in the truest sense of those terms? Therefore, the questions remain unanswered: Who will appeal for consequences? Who will appeal for rights? Who will appeal for virtues? Who will appeal for justice and equality? And to whom? After working as a medical practitioner for nearly two decades in an enormously populated country, India, at the grassroots level, I faced these challenges repeatedly. These challenges were awful, especially in the context of my dual role as a clinician and an informal caregiver while taking care of my mother, who has dementia. I felt this dilemma in every step and have realized that this systemic malfunction is global. The same size does not fit all. There are various senses of justice, and we need to identify those case by case. It seems the overarching classical triad of depression, i.e., loneliness, boredom, and helplessness, somehow restricts clinicians from acting as social purifiers; however, this is a must to prevent the growing concern of the general population toward a therapeutic nihilism.

In the United States, mainly due to Social Security benefits, implementation of various health policies, and increased life expectancy, the status of older adults is now considered an "advantaged" category (Hudson & Gonyea, 2012). However, the situation is changing dramatically and needs some drastic actions to implement new policies. Otherwise, a considerable portion of older adults will continue to be considered "contenders" and continue fighting to keep their social status the same. In contrast, vulnerable others may be downgraded back to the "dependent status," seeking health programs targeted to assist them. These upcoming challenges are considered moral, social, and legal threats to elders (McCullough, 2000). The resultant may be a social concern; it may give rise to distinct stratifications of aging cohorts in the society, and then…?

2.2 Bioethics and Medicalization

The latest advancements in medicine have increased longevity across the globe (Singh, 2010). However, how is the current quality of life in those extra gained days due to the blessings of medicalization? How honest are the clinicians, in this respect, while taking care of the diseased? The "Introduction" of the book *Being Mortal* by Dr. Atul Gawande (2014) is a fluent discussion of various aspects of mortality from a clinician's point of view that reflects a more humanistic and less medicalized approach to death and dying. According to Dr. Gawande, there may be some unrecognized, but still prevalent, ideas that we never thought of before; we must pick up those in the management of terminal illnesses. Dr. Gawande has tried to compare the later life in a developed country, where he is practicing, with a developing one, where his origin was. The author is entirely successful in his intention in describing the conflicts between wanting to employ the most effective medical procedures and the need to address the humanistic elements of the dying experience for the patient and the family. The examples are so vivid as if they were our next-door neighbor. On the one hand, the characters are from a country (the United States) where personal liberty is a fundamental right. On the other hand, the figures from another country (India) depict a scenario where traditionalism is the mainstay of life.

Even after practicing as a surgeon for decades in a developed country, Dr. Gawande is still searching for meaningful satisfaction in his profession. According to him, "we paid our medical tuition to learn about the inner process of the body, the intricate mechanisms of its pathologies, and the vast trove of discoveries and technologies that have accumulated to stop them. We did not imagine we needed to think about much else" (Gawande, 2014, p. 3). The experiences are reminiscent of my position as a practicing family physician back in India, where most of my care recipients were of the "older adult" age group. This lookout for emotional satisfaction was intense as a practitioner in a developing country where the population is humongous and the patient-doctor ratio is much higher. Therefore, often the work becomes monotonous, which satisfies neither the patients nor the clinicians. If a doctor needs to work for 48 hours without any break, the concept (or imagination!) of achieving mental satisfaction becomes a luxury there. Therefore, the treatment becomes synonymous with only prescribing some medicines due to a lack of psychological bonding from both doctor and patient. Also, no new conceptions regarding the management of chronic diseases arise in the doctors' minds. As a consequence, corruption intervenes through this hole. This gap is not a fault of either of the persons concerned, though both become sufferers. Any feeling related to morbidity and mortality should be equally shared between the healthcare provider and the concerned patients and their close family members, but a variable degree of overlap may exist between the interests of the patient and doctor (Dorr Goold & Lipkin, 1999). However, practically, this relationship is in a violent situation in the present socioeconomic circumstances anywhere in the world.

I can remember that night, over 20 years ago, when I was an intern in the medicine department and was treating my first "official" patient at midnight. A patient with chronic obstructive pulmonary disease in his late 70s was almost in a gasping condition. However, an aminophylline drip worked like magic; within half an hour, he felt better and started talking. It was an unbelievable situation for me after helping the patient without any assistance from senior physicians. This kind of incident, i.e., independent handling of the patients, happened again and again. I was surprised by my own work and started thinking about various prospects. Nevertheless, slowly, I realized I got stuck in this profession—to fulfill some personal demands, family demands, demands of plenty of care recipients, representatives of various pharmaceutical companies and diagnostic centers, and many others not in these categories. The heroic attitude gradually changed into an acerbic one.

Dr. Gawande also has mentioned that the primary responsibilities of a medical doctor are honesty and kindness. We, the doctors, often forget those things while working, either in the hospital or at private clinics. The medical profession is one of the noblest ones. However, very few physicians/surgeons consider themselves as healthcare providers from this perspective. In the era of the "Consumer Protection Act," this profession is only *one* among many others where we find ourselves as moneymaking machines. We tend to snatch from people as much as possible from this profession for ourselves and our nuclear families. Humanity becomes secondary here.

Honesty can be interpreted from different dimensions, but we are not in any means truthful to our oaths, which we had taken at the time of graduation from medical school. Dr. Gawande is right; we are inflicting new forms of physical (and mental) torture on our patients while practicing as a modern-day therapist. While searching for the answer to the question, "who are the primitive ones?," Dr. Gawande was also wondering. Therefore, the significance of the modern day's medical improvements remains unanswered. Though it may sound ridiculous, I am, in fact, still wondering what exactly I want to do in the future. Every physician prefers to do something that will put a smile on their face and the faces of those they are assisting. Moreover, now, it is an obvious realization that I must do something different so that I can at least recognize the various meanings of different smiles. However, honesty is like memory, hard to measure precisely, and sometimes looks different in retrospect. Therefore, at the same time, after successfully practicing as an honest (I have a doubt now!) physician, now I want to run away from my profession; I do not wish to practice further as a clinician. It is still unclear since when I have started feeling this way. Has this feeling grown stronger during the time of not practicing? Nevertheless, this is a strong feeling that perhaps I am the misfit, …misfit in the surrounding environment.

In the book *Hospital Land USA*, Dr. Wendy Simonds (2017) narrated plenty of the emotional experiences she had at different ages during her presence in the hospital lands. But all those are either as a patient or as a patient's companion. I have experience as a patient, patient companion, as well as a service provider (physician). Somehow, the experiences are similar in all the roles, either as a care provider or a care recipient. Though hospital land is a peculiar coexistence of joy and sorrow, many more people are getting positive results from the land of hospitals. Still, many times, a fear of impending loss (death!) prevailed in my mind. Those memories are terrifying to me. The author also narrated this experience in her nighttime adventures (Simonds, 2017, p. 94). I wonder whether my feelings arise from a fear of sins that I committed as a care provider or as a care recipient after receiving unsatisfactory care. At least obstetrician Dr. "A" waited for (two decades ago) 1 hour for a particular baby to be delivered, while now many doctors do not spend even moments for "birth from below" (Simonds, 2017). Scissors and knife-blades are more "comfortable" in every aspect, and the future and well-being of the mother (patient!) is not a matter of concern. It seems like every possible way of healthy survival, at this moment, is equally hopeless and realistic—an exhaustion within satire, a cry inside laughter. Long corridors of any hospital land may be described as "road to heaven," "tunnel of anxiety," "way of life," "path of destruction," or "path of rebirth," by different persons, but by any means, no one wants to return to that corridor again. Dr. Simonds realized that some patients do not have time for doctor shopping. If everyone has time, could they still manage to find their doctor of choice? Still unsure, but after going through this book, this was the first realization that we were, probably, in a world of fantasy regarding the health system of a so-called developed country. After realizing the contemporary medical cost, it is a real panic now, especially in a situation where it could be hard even to afford the medical insurance cost of a nuclear family.

In this era of medicalization, regarding the usage of the terms "patient" versus "client," this has been an ongoing debate in the clinical field, especially in mental health circles, for many years. The term "client" is more often used by those who consider themselves humanistic and want to break down the personal barrier between "doctor" and "patient." On the other hand, the term "patient" implies an illness and is more often used in medical circles. Many psychologists believe that in order to ultimately provide (and be reimbursed for) non-pharmacological services to those with mental health problems, we have to adopt medical terminology (V. Molinari, personal communication, October 16, 2020). In this regard, another question that comes to mind is about doctor shopping. What happens when a depressed patient/client visits a clinician who is actually more depressed? One of the general competencies for all psychologists/clinicians is professional values and attitudes. Clinicians need to monitor themselves to make sure they are in good mental health so as not to "infect" patients. Clinicians are considered practicing "outside of their competence" if they are depressed and unable to help those who are paying them for mental/physical health services (V. Molinari, personal communication, October 8, 2020). However, in real-life situations, how is professional dignity maintained in this relationship? Who would judge this? Does a patient or their family members ever judge a clinician based on their level of depression? Perhaps, still, this consideration depends on their degree of professionalism. The actuality remains hidden by convention. Although our aim is to find newer techniques to attract more "clients," the interest of "patients" always remains secondary.

The influence of medicalization in our lives (especially concerning end-of-life experiences) is gradually becoming increasingly significant. The modern treatment protocol has extended the life span of human beings by at least 5–7 years than what it was three or four decades ago. Thus, medicalization is emerging as a social problem and increasing day by day. We are now confused about whether medicalization is a blessing or a curse for end-of-life care. The present stifling condition of medicalization does not allow us to breathe properly. In the last few decades, the basic patterns of health and morbidity are continually changing. Many regular life events, such as birth, death, menarche, menopause, and aging, are now considered medical problems. Medicalization is spreading like a black shadow over all these natural life events.

However, we are from a country where "service (care) for souls without expectation" is given maximum importance and is continuing since ancient times. Terms like industrialization, urbanization, and globalization are making our lives more complicated. To achieve a larger quantity of life, we are losing the quality of life. I believe everything is predetermined, and one will just receive their lot. Doctors are only part of a system; blaming the doctors is nothing but an expression of our frustration in life. The traditional Indian societal model has excellent concepts regarding the all-around development of an individual (Tiwari & Pandey, 2013). This concept can make us calm and stable and help us to gain satisfaction in our lives. However, today's India is not that what I am talking about. Unfortunately, we are declining in almost every domain of morality. Many Western societies are attracted to Eastern cultures; however, our traditional societal model is gradually going into oblivion due to our blind and inappropriate imitation of Western culture. These thoughts are significant in the discussion of the current issue of the doctor-patient relationship.

In the first few days as a resident house physician in the oncology ward, we had to follow Dr. Ganguly (name changed), the senior of our two visiting professors. During the patient visit (ward round), I often tried to take him first to the bed of the patient who died the night before or on that morning. He frequently reminded us of our inability to do something with these terminal patients and that they just come to the hospital to die, and since it was not my fault, I do not need to worry about those incidents. This assurance from a senior professor gradually increased our confidence during those days until another visiting professor, Dr. Mukherjee (name changed), came back from his leave. I used the same "formula" and suddenly realized how angry he was with my attitude. Dr. Mukherjee was just the opposite of the other visiting professor. He blamed me for any patient's death in that ward (we, each resident physician, had to take responsibility for a whole different ward). According to him, being a resident physician for this entire ward, I was the only culprit. He taught me that as a resident physician, I must stay in the ward not only during duty hours but also beyond that, if possible, for 24 hours. He made us realize that this was not only a physician's duty but also a moral responsibility. Patients come to the hospital not to die but to survive. Within a few days, I started forgetting to take him toward the beds of "just-died" patients. I do not know how efficient I am now as a physician, but those attitudes in the first months of training had changed my entire outlook for the future. A common notion is that doctors belong to one of the higher layers of the education system in every society; this is not only because they are intelligent and diligent but also because they prepare themselves for the role of acting as a bridge between life and death. For doctors, it required thousands of years to achieve this level of trust in society. Therefore, if we, the doctors, remain honest in our profession, we can make a new world of hope, and, indeed, Dr. Gawande will consider a revision of his "Introduction" chapter in *Being Mortal*.

Primary care doctors often overlook the minute symptoms and signs, particularly in the diagnosis of mental illness. Even after the diagnosis, the "ego" to work collaboratively with the other paramedical workers acts as a negative factor regarding the treatment. I experienced these situations several times in my country, India. This attitude is also a global problem, though doctors are not solely responsible for this negligence. Instead, the busy life and the introduction of the "Consumer Protection Act" prevent building a healthy doctor-patient relationship there in the present-day, which was not common even a couple of decades ago. In our childhood, even a few years back, there were plenty of family physicians who used to treat every disease, at least for the first few days. They knew "everything" about the concerned family members, even many personal issues that were unrelated to the disease. There was much respect in that doctor-patient relationship from either end. Nowadays, there are ample specialists in different branches of medicine and surgery. People consult them even on the initial days of a particular illness, not knowing them personally, just looking at their degrees. However, the medical diagnosis does not depend only on the "degrees" of the concerned physician. Sometimes patients consider this attitude as a status symbol or sometimes do not rely on the knowledge of the family physicians, and somehow humanity is replaced by technology and a professional approach. Now, most doctors do not have much time for their patients. We, the doctors, do not always remain sincere to our professional ethics and often forget about the oath we took at the time of receiving our medical degrees. Therefore, the problems often remain unrecognized and undertreated, especially when the concerned patient is an older person and the disease is related to mental health. We need to be engrossed in listening to them and make the environment more relaxing, where the older adults could feel comfortable talking to us. Paying attention to them is the only way to earn trust and respect.

Here I want to mention an aged person who not only surprised us but also helped numerous other people in society. He, Dr. Shibsundar Bhattacharyya (name changed), was our family physician in India. Even in his late 80s, he was disciplined and accurate, both in lifestyle and efficiency as a clinician, with hearing aids and high-power glass on his eyes. The tremendous workload he took on his shoulder as a family physician mesmerized everyone. He definitely developed some compensatory mechanisms during his work schedules, but he never became annoyed with his patients, and his patients always depended on him until his last day. This dependency, which I realized after becoming a doctor, helped him a lot to find motivation in his monotonous work and helped in his longevity. Even though he died on a patient's shoulder while examining him, after he expired many witnessed his patients' heartbreaking cries; many of them even came from a distance only to show their final respect for him. I cannot imagine myself getting such respect from my patients.

At this point of discussion, anyone may assume that the doctors are the greediest in the current world. Definitely, the intention is not to focus on that. Instead, this profession is like the backbone of any society, and the majority of doctors is honest, which is why everything is going so smoothly in our surrounding health sector. The current COVID-19 pandemic has shown how physicians are leading the caregiving sector. Many doctors nearly sacrificed their life for a broader social benefit. Dishonesty is interfering in every profession, everywhere now, though exceptions still exist. Fortunately, these exceptions are still much more in number than their negative counterparts, and collectively for those exceptions, we are moving forward. The physicians have to survive in this leading role in making a change for society. As this profession is closely related to life and death, anything abnormal comes under autopsy. However, the current pandemic has reminded the entire world that physicians are still the last hope through their leadership roles, their humanity, and their invincible determination. The role of physicians could be viewed from a different perspective during this unprecedented time. Currently, we are facing a massive shortage of healthcare professionals globally. At this point in time, there must be some flexibility, at least for the physicians who are treating numerous helpless persons with a critical need for a healthy life. If an Indian physician can treat an American in India, then why can he not treat an Indian in America or vice versa? Practicing licensure in any country must not be a barrier for the physicians who received a medical degree from a different country to treat persons with disorders. If an academic can work without the bindings of international licensure, then why not a physician? There should be a consensus at the international level; the World Health Organization should play a pivotal role in this matter.

2.3 Conclusion

As all medical conditions are not covered under insurance policies, the cost of healthcare is growing out of reach with each passing day, and many businessmen are invading the medical arena only for profit without having any basic knowledge of medical science. Therefore, this noble profession of physician no longer remains noble now. All these domains are interconnected, and gradually we are losing discipline in every field. Therefore, a revolutionary approach must come from every honest (and those who want to be honest but are victimized in the current system) person of this globe to establish a disciplined system across the world. Otherwise, we cannot protect our civilization from evils. Dishonesty will defeat humanity. In this war, our elderly generation can play a significant role through their experience and wisdom. Nonetheless, we should progress forward to implement some new policies in this regard because we, by any means, want not to move out of our focus to give our older adult population a productive life, at least for our benefit.

References

Das, S. (2019). *Legalising passive euthanasia in India: Ethical & legal challenges after common cause judgement.* Retrieved on October 19, 2020. Available at: https://papers.ssrn.com/sol3/papers.cfm?abstract_id=3503792

Dorr Goold, S., & Lipkin, M., Jr. (1999). The doctor-patient relationship: Challenges, opportunities, and strategies. *Journal of General Internal Medicine, 14*(Suppl 1), S26–S33. https://doi.org/10.1046/j.1525-1497.1999.00267.x

Drossman, D. A., & Ruddy, J. (2021). *Gut feelings: Disorders of gut-brain interaction and the patient-doctor relationship.* Drossman Care.

Gawande, A. (2014). *Being mortal. Medicine and what matters most in the end*. Metropolitan Press. ISBN: 978-1410478122.

Hudson, R. B., & Gonyea, J. G. (2012). Baby boomers and the shifting political construction of old age. *The Gerontologist, 52*(2), 272–282. https://doi.org/10.1093/geront/gnr129

Mandal, J., Ponnambath, D. K., & Parija, S. C. (2016). Utilitarian and deontological ethics in medicine. *Tropical Parasitology, 6*(1), 5–7. https://doi.org/10.4103/2229-5070.175024

McCullough, L. (2000). Bioethics and aging. In T. Cole, R. Kastenbaum, & R. Ray (Eds.), *Handbook of the humanities and aging* (pp. 93–113). Springer Publishing Company.

Pappas, G., Kiriaze, I. J., & Falagas, M. E. (2008). Insights into infectious disease in the era of Hippocrates. *International Journal of Infectious Diseases, 12*(4), 347–350. https://doi.org/10.1016/j.ijid.2007.11.003

Raus, K., Mortier, E., & Eeckloo, K. (2018). The patient perspective in health care networks. *BMC Medical Ethics, 19*(1), 52. https://doi.org/10.1186/s12910-018-0298-x

Simonds, W. (2017). *Hospital land USA: Sociological adventures in medicalization*. Routledge.

Sims, J. M. (2010). A brief review of the Belmont report. *Dimensions of Critical Care Nursing: DCCN, 29*(4), 173–174. https://doi.org/10.1097/DCC.0b013e3181de9ec5

Singh, A. R. (2010). Modern medicine: Towards prevention, cure, well-being and longevity. *Mens Sana Monographs, 8*(1), 17–29. https://doi.org/10.4103/0973-1229.58817

Tiwari, S. C., & Pandey, N. M. (2013). The Indian concepts of lifestyle and mental health in old age. *Indian Journal of Psychiatry, 55*(Suppl S2), 288–292.

Chapter 3
Aging and Retirement

3.1 Retirement: A Blessing or a Curse

Work is probably the most crucial social engagement of every adult person. On the other hand, *retirement* is the action of leaving one's job or work after reaching a certain age. As the population is "graying" throughout the globe, the term "retirement" is gaining importance day by day from different newer perspectives. It is probably one of the inevitable destinations of every human adult, and it regulates an intergenerational social cycle that operates the status of the economic development of a country. As the world progresses, today's aging population has more options regarding retirement planning from work that were never present before. Retirement is considered a milestone in an individual's life. Although the concerned person knows that they are logically retiring from work only, not from life, in reality, it does not always feel like that. That is why many people think of it as a curse, not a blessing. This mindset influences individuals' cognitive function and overall health. Ekerdt (2010) advocates for an individualized approach; he considered that personality traits might endorse it. For some, retirement is a sense of relief from monotonous activities; even they may want to retire early. However, for many, retirement is a curse; for those of pensionable age who cannot afford to retire but cannot continue working because of poor health, aging parents who need care, potential employers would rather hire younger workers. In contrast, one may feel unhappy only because of a lack of "busy-ness" (Ekerdt, 2010). It is very common to feel lost, scared, or sad when approaching this important milestone; these individuals may want to retire late or at least want to be self-employed part-time.

My father-in-law, Mr. Santanu Bhattacharya, a mechanical engineer by profession, felt a negativity within himself during the later years of service in a government institution. That time he worked in an environment surrounded by junior employees and thought they are not giving proper respect to him. This feeling developed an ego problem, which compelled him to take voluntary retirement from his job. However, soon after leaving his job, he realized that it was not the right decision. Because at that time, there were not enough things in his hands to be engaged. He felt that motivation is not always essential; instead, engagement is necessary regarding passing the time, especially at this age. Gradually he became depressed and desperately started doing something to be engaged but felt that it was not of his standard by any means. His depression persisted until he got another job 3 years later in his domain. He was lucky to manage at least a part-time job a few years after his retirement; everyone does not get that opportunity, and retirement becomes a curse for them.

There is an interrelationship between work and retirement that always persists in the context of aging from a multidisciplinary perspective. Aging is usually negatively stereotyped as less productive, less trainable, and less promotable (Diekman & Hirnisey, 2007). Often, employers are reluctant to employ older adults because they are expensive, especially when companies need to cover parts of their health insurance (Staudinger et al., 2016); however, this is not always true. According to Wang and Shi (2016), work gives us income, social security, personal autonomy, and fame. As we progress toward our old age, our relationship with the concerned organization plays a vital role in our withdrawal (self-imposed or forced) from the organization. Although our cognitive impairments commonly manifest as we progress toward old age, our experiences and expertise still increase. Therefore, for maintaining a good relationship, we try to perform better and better (in terms of loyalty and productivity) for the benefit of our organization and reciprocally receive benefits (economic, health, or socio-emotional) from the organization. This relationship is also true in the context of human resource management. Older workers feel most comfortable with their job security in terms of physical, economic, and proper opportunities to use their skills. This group of employees feels more comfortable in their job settings to mentor others, stay motivated with challenging jobs with flexible hours, and maintain a good relationship with the management. However, the most influential factor in an employee's productivity is maintaining a proper balance between work and family demands, which ultimately leads to severe stress in employees. Workplace policies should allow employees to access paid time off to participate in physical activities or mindfulness programs to reduce this kind of stress in older workers (Pitt-Catsouphes et al., 2015). Policy implications should motivate employers to hire older workers and utilize their skills at the highest possible level by providing them job security and satisfaction. In the context of the present world, in the transition from work to retirement life, "the temporal model" of retirement is gradually gaining increasing importance, which suggests three distinct phases of this transition, namely. Planning for retirement, decision-making, and postretirement adjustments in life (Wang & Shi, 2016). This transition controls the well-being of the concerned person remarkably economically, physically, and psychologically. In later life, all these issues profoundly impact the morbidity and life span of the individual. This transitional phase is also a multidisciplinary area and requires more longitudinal research to better understand the interventions from a global perspective.

3.2   Retirement: Theoretical Perspectives

There are different age-related changes in an individual's life course, which affect the work motivation in middle-aged and older adult workers from a theoretical perspective (Kanfer & Ackerman, 2004). According to Kanfer and Ackerman (2004), certain abilities reach their maximum at different ages, such as fluid intellectual ability (associated with cognitive skills and working memory) in younger ages and crystalline intellectual ability (those achieved through education and experience) in later life. Regarding personality traits, some of those decline as we age (like openness), and some increase (like conscientiousness). In old age, greater use of self-control, self-concept, and identity development influence an individual's motivational outcomes. In general, we assume that older workers are less motivated, but interindividual differences exist across the life course. In this context, Kanfer's model of motivational processing is very significant. This model shows how to promote positive effects toward work motivation by way of organizational strategies (Kanfer & Ackerman, 2004) like rewarding intrinsic (such as improving training or learning measures) or extrinsic (such as offering incentives, promotion, or lucrative pension schemes) manner (Staudinger et al., 2016). Therefore, policy modifications should encourage employers to provide older workers with the best possible environment to maximize their productivity. Furthermore, in many low-income countries, older workers' working ability needs to be protected by some sort of social security benefits to minimize their economic and physical frailty.

The selection, optimization, and compensation (SOC) model (Baltes & Baltes, 1990) has gained more importance in the work context in the past decades. Research suggests that the application of SOC strategy has a significant positive association with age, job autonomy, self-reported and non-self-reported job performance, job satisfaction, and job engagement (Moghimi et al., 2017). However, SOC strategy is not highly associated with job tenure, job demands, and job strain (Moghimi et al., 2017). Weigl et al. (2013) described workability as the employees' capability to perform their work concerning physical and psychological job demands. They found a three-way interaction effect of age, job control, and SOC strategies on workability. On the other hand, Baltes (1993) argued that the aging mind needs to be considered a concept of an equilibrium of potential and limits. This opinion is more acceptable because there is a substantial interference of the cognitive mechanics by biological-genetic-health factors, and decline with aging is likely (Baltes, 1993).

There is enough evidence that the association between retirement and health status, including cognitive functioning, especially in older adults, is bidirectional, i.e., both having a direct impact on the other (Wu et al., 2016). A wide body of literature examined the association between retirement age and longevity, revealing mixed findings (Wu et al., 2016). Analyzing data of 2956 participants from the Health and Retirement Study, Wu and colleagues (2016) found that early retirement may hasten time to death and prolonged working life may provide survival benefits among US adults. Also, it is evident that the association between retirement and cognitive decline is affected by the characteristics of the person's occupation (Meng et al., 2017). Meng et al. (2017) found an association between retirement and cognitive functioning, and the rate of cognitive decline varies between jobs having different levels of mental demands. They suggested that in individuals retiring from jobs high in complexity, retirement expedites the rate of decline in crystallized cognitive abilities. However, the effect of retirement on the rate of decline in fluid cognitive abilities is conflicting. To date, there is still a considerable research gap existing in this domain, especially in the context of conflicting theories. According to the "use it or lose it" theory, an individual may experience sudden cognitive decline postretirement due to the abrupt reduction of mentally challenging works. In contrast, the "cognitive reserve" theory proposes that an individual can escape from sudden postretirement cognitive deterioration only due to having a better cognitive reserve, i.e., having the ability to use neural networks more efficiently than others. Also, we need to know how personality traits influence the association between retirement and cognitive functioning. However, what happens if there is job satisfaction? To date, we have no idea about how multiple jobs (in different occupational fields)/"re-retirements" (consecutive retirements) in midlife affect cognitive performance in old age and how long the effects persist. The impact of work and retirement on elderly workers' perceptions of health is considered a strong predictor of morbidity and mortality. Celidoni et al. (2017) found that retirement has a long-term deleterious effect on cognitive performance for individuals nearing retirement age. Though some retire on a near-retirement scheme, early retirement plays a protective role in their well-being. A study by Westerlund et al. (2009) revealed that high physical and psychological job demands and low job satisfaction in older workers were associated with a steep increase in suboptimum health before retirement and increased benefits from retirement. The findings suggest that the burden of poor health in terms of perceived health problems in older workers with poor working conditions is greatly relieved by retirement. Nevertheless, the retirement-related health benefit was more related to work than to private life.

It is evident that physical activity, intellectual activity, and many lifestyle factors associated with the work environment could impact age-related physical and mental changes (Staudinger et al., 2016). For many, these cumulative adverse life experiences challenge their survival (Banerjee & Duflo, 2007), with minimal effect on the work environment, thus supporting Ekerdt's (2010) views. Tailoring retirement age to the specific needs of the older person would be the best possible solution. Therefore, an individualized approach, including the level of job demand, job satisfaction, perceived health status of individuals, and postretirement (institutional) benefits as the most important factors, needs to be considered before deciding on a more encompassing retirement policy that may be best applied population wide.

3.3   Retirement and Intergenerational Relationships

From my professional dealings, I have seen many individuals while in their working life, enjoying (or in frustration with) their retirement life, or anxious about their future while in the transition phase. However, the most influential example I experienced in my personal life is with my parents, who even in their early 70s lived in a separate house isolated from their offspring. My father, the late Mr. Kalyan Bhattacharyya, was economically secure, previously with his government job and after retirement with his pension. He was a government employee for 42 years at the same institution (though in different posts and with several promotions from 18 to up to 60 years of age). He was on a monthly salary, and after retirement he got various benefits (like provident fund, gratuity, and lifelong monthly pension) from his workplace. He was very egoistic and possessed much power in his family and wanted to control it forever. He did not take anything which comes from his son's income. During the later years of his job, he became less motivated due to his public service's monotonous nature. Still, he was engaged in his job to enjoy full retirement benefits. However, a few weeks after retirement, he again became frustrated thinking about how to pass the time. His physical and mental health gradually started declining. However, when my mother started showing the manifestations of dementia and she needed every assistance in her daily basic activities, my father provided all those supports. Although my father never played the role as a caregiver in our family in his working life, he was engaged in that new job and did that with pleasure. My father was anxious about their future but no longer frustrated about how to pass the time. Still, they were not willing to take any support from their children. In my opinion, they thought it would diminish their image, in front of others. I do not know; they might have had more expectations from their son that I could not fulfill. I was busy with my profession and my lifestyle in this materialistic world. Therefore, I never noticed the gradual progression of this generation gap. In the last few years, I noticed that they were even refusing to take medical advice from me; they were visiting our family physician uncle, who used to treat us before I became a doctor. Now I am in a different country, and this relocation may not be solely from my passion for *dementia*; there might be a subtle connection with the fact that I also wanted to run away from my place, from my country, and from my profession myself. I did not want to practice further. I wanted to change my present profession, with which I cannot assist my mother. After successfully practicing as a dedicated physician for nearly two decades, I do not know what exactly my future focus is on gerontology. We are *dying* (crushing) in every moment, every day in our real-life situation, and the *loss* we experience through this is no less than real *death*. To some extent, all these are closely related to my new journey, in search of eternal satisfaction, to find positivity from an apparent gloomy atmosphere.

A turbulent relationship between two successive generations is ubiquitous in today's family life. For many older adults, retirement is a blessing; after years of following other peoples' rules, they expect a sense of relief when they want to live their lives by their rules. However, the subtle idea of retirement should not be entangled only by the transition from pre-older adults to older adults on a specific day; instead, this transitioning occurs in every day, every moment, even beyond that age. Many older adults do not wish to accept any help even from their children due to a sense of losing independence in their lives (Brody, 2010; Laditka, 2017). Therefore, my parents are not unusual from a global perspective. Often the victims are of the sandwich generation, who felt stress and guilt in every phase of their life. Due to urbanization and the current socioeconomic situation, many individuals have to become long-distance caretakers for their parents. For some, this transition is by choice, as they did not ask for help. In my opinion, an ego clash is responsible for this turbulence, a transition from extended family to nuclear family, due to psycho-social causes. Extending a hand is not only a responsibility of the younger generation, but the younger generation also expects the same from the older one. They need to realize that the current world is rushing, the pace is faster than ever, and space is limited, so a family should proceed in every step like a *family*, not as an individual.

Ageism is a big issue in this context. Ageism is the idea of stereotyping or discrimination against an individual based on their age. While discussing different social or public health concerns, we often remark that education is crucial in realizing the concerned issue better from a practical standpoint. We always focus on the beneficial roles of education and the quality of the way it is delivered; however, we never think about the quality of its contents. From the beginning, a child is taught that "young" or "modern" is the opposite word of "old." At their age, children often cannot recognize what is wrong or right; they only learn whatever they are being taught. Every one of us was a child once upon a time, and till the last day of our lives, the mirror of our mind will reflect what we learned at the elementary school level. We can never get rid of the image that an older person is the opposite of a young or modern person. Therefore, in our perception, an older adult can never be young or modern, both physically and mentally. Ageism invades through this whole. I have a strong objection here. I always argue for the reconsideration of our thought process regarding the relationship between two generations. We never think in a way that aging is a natural process and that old is complementing young, not opposing, in the same way as we learned that "day" is the opposite of "night," "man" is the opposite of "woman," "black" is the opposite of "white," and "mother" is the opposite of "father." Is it so? Is this a flaw of our education system itself or our wrong input in the contents of the education system? We need to update our education system first. We need to change our thought process that opposite words are not always opposing each other; instead, they complement each other in most cases. We can label a profession based on the purpose of work it serves but cannot prejudice an individual based only on that label. Otherwise, it will be a further challenge for us to show dignity to others, our forefathers, and the relationship between the two generations will always remain tumultuous.

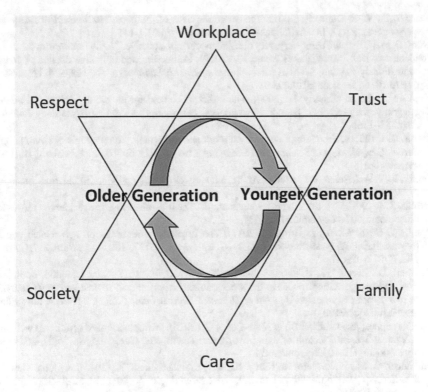

Fig. 3.1 Complementary theory of aging

3.4 Conclusion

We are retiring from many events in our everyday life, intentionally or unintentionally. Wrinkles of skin, graying of hair, or cognitive declines are only part of some physiological processes. A complementary relationship is a must to ease our journey. This "complementary theory of aging" (as shown in Fig. 3.1) has the potential to harmonize the entire concept of aging. When we will realize this journey, the purpose of our education will be successful. Ageism will no longer exist then, and the question of whether retirement is a curse or blessing will disappear itself.

References

Baltes, P. B. (1993). The aging mind: Potential and limits. *The Gerontologist, 33*(5), 580–594. https://doi.org/10.1093/geront/33.5.580

Baltes, P. B., & Baltes, M. M. (1990). Psychological perspectives on successful aging: The model of selective optimization with compensation. In P. B. Baltes & M. M. Baltes (Eds.), *Successful aging: Perspectives from the behavioral sciences* (pp. 1–34). Cambridge University Press.

Banerjee, A. V., & Duflo, E. (2007). The economic lives of the poor. *The Journal of Economic Perspectives, 21*(1), 141–167. https://doi.org/10.1257/jep.21.1.141

Brody, E. M. (2010). On being very, very old: An insider's perspective. *The Gerontologist, 50*, 2–10.

Celidoni, M., Dal Bianco, C., & Weber, G. (2017). Retirement and cognitive decline. A longitudinal analysis using SHARE data. *Journal of Health Economics, 56*, 113–125. https://doi.org/10.1016/j.jhealeco.2017.09.003

Diekman, A. B., & Hirnisey, L. (2007). The effect of context on the silvery ceiling: A role of congruity perspective on prejudiced responses. *Personality and Social Psychology Bulletin, 33*, 1353–1366.

Ekerdt, D. J. (2010). Frontiers of research on work and retirement. *The Journals of Gerontology. Series B, Psychological Sciences and Social Sciences, 65B*(1), 69–80. https://doi.org/10.1093/geronb/gbp109

Kanfer, R., & Ackerman, P. L. (2004). Aging, adult development, and work motivation. *Academy of Management Review, 29*, 440–458.

Laditka, S. B. (2017). "It can't happen soon enough." The role of readiness in residential moves by older parents. *The Gerontologist, 57*(1), 6–11.

Meng, A., Nexø, M. A., & Borg, V. (2017). The impact of retirement on age related cognitive decline – A systematic review. *BMC Geriatrics, 17*(1), 160. https://doi.org/10.1186/s12877-017-0556-7

Moghimi, D., Zacher, H., Scheibe, S., & Van Yperen, N. W. (2017). The selection, optimization, and compensation model in the work context: A systematic review and meta-analysis of two decades of research. *Journal of Organizational Behavior, 38*(2), 247–275. https://doi.org/10.1002/job.2108

Pitt-Catsouphes, M., James, J. B., & Matz-Costa, C. (2015). Workplace-based health and wellness programs: The intersection of aging, work, and health. *The Gerontologist, 55*(2), 262–270. https://doi.org/10.1093/geront/gnu114

Staudinger, U. M., Finkelstein, R., Calvo, E., & Sivaramakrishnan, K. (2016). A global view on the effects of work on health in later life. *The Gerontologist, 56*(Suppl 2), S281–S292. https://doi.org/10.1093/geront/gnw032

Wang, M., & Shi, J. (2016). Work, retirement, and aging. In K. W. Schaie & S. L. Willis (Eds.), *Handbook of psychology of aging* (8th ed., pp. 339–356). Academic Press.

Weigl, M., Müller, A., Hornung, S., Zacher, H., & Angerer, P. (2013). The moderating effects of job control and selection, optimization, and compensation strategies on the age-work ability relationship. *Journal of Organizational Behavior, 34*(5), 607–628. https://doi.org/10.1002/job.1810

Westerlund, H., Kivimaki, M., Singh-Manoux, A., Melchior, M., Ferrie, J. E., Pentti, J., Jokela, M., Leineweber, C., Goldberg, M., Zins, M., & Vahtera, J. (2009). Self-rated health before and after retirement in France (GAZEL): A cohort study. *Lancet, 374*(9705), 1889–1896.

Wu, C., Odden, M. C., Fisher, G. G., & Stawski, R. S. (2016). Association of retirement age with mortality: A population-based longitudinal study among older adults in the USA. *Journal of Epidemiology and Community Health, 70*(9), 917–923. https://doi.org/10.1136/jech-2015-207097.

Chapter 4
Healthy Aging and Aging Well

4.1 Promoting Concepts of Better Aging or Aging Well

As the global population is graying, the term "healthy aging" is gradually emerging as one of the most significant phrases in the current world of caregiving. Different determinants influence the outcome of aging in various stages of our life course. In a literature review, "Investing in Health…," Fried discussed that the full benefits of an aging society would be achieved if elderly people stay healthy and can stay engaged in any roles that contribute to societal benefits (Fried, 2016). In any discussion regarding healthy aging, the doctor-patient relationship comes up undoubtedly. Whether it is primary, secondary, and tertiary care or prevention and health promotion, the mainstay is the same everywhere. According to Fried (2016), some chronic diseases, such as stroke, chronic obstructive pulmonary diseases, and diabetes, cause higher disability rates for older adults of developing countries than those of developed ones. In my opinion, these older adults are practically burdened to their family members, particularly in the socioeconomic structure of developing countries like India. Currently, there is no significant social welfare program in India that offers assistance to these seniors. The only response to their emergency health problems seems to be hospitalization. Most of them feel neglected, both in their family and society. They have found themselves very lonely in the surrounding world (Singh & Misra, 2009). These are, to some extent, due to their reduction in work efficiency, declination in earning capacity, suffering from different chronic diseases, memory loss, an increasing number of nuclear families, and as a consequence, gradual communication problems with the next generation. A large number of older adults are holding on to the hope of achieving healthy aging, but the resources are limited. As mentioned earlier, there is a profuse shortage of clinicians; adding to that there is also a dearth of other resource persons who can guide them toward healthy aging. Even the term *gerontology* itself is relatively uncommon in India.

© The Author(s), under exclusive license to Springer Nature Switzerland AG 2021   23
K. K. Bhattacharyya, *Rethinking the Aging Transition*,
https://doi.org/10.1007/978-3-030-88870-1_4

The world is moving very fast. At a similar pace, the concept of healthy aging also is constantly changing. The ideas that were considered acceptable a few years ago are no longer valid today. The concept differs across the cultures with a great amount of inter- and intrapersonal variations. The Western world has thrown the ideas of the extended intergenerational family since long days back, and the Eastern world is rushing toward that culture today. Many community-dwelling older adults currently have multiple living options, from various old age communities to isolated and autonomous living, from living as a member of an extended multigenerational family to living in a nuclear family. The choice entirely depends on the concerned individual according to the situation. However, for many others, the option is considered a luxury. Therefore, the experience of healthy aging differs in many ways. The experience of liberty and control gives a joyous feeling one day, and on another it shows a "boomerang" effect. Modernization will persist forever, and the impact of the increase in the human life span will depend on how we (not only the older adults) can adapt to the situations. We will be able to proceed a step ahead toward aging better only after this adaptation takes place with a universal acceptance.

The current idea of healthy aging, as directed by the World Health Organization (WHO), emphasizes "the process of developing and maintaining the functional ability that enables wellbeing in older age" (World Health Organization, 2020). Healthy aging is the focus of the WHO's projects on older adults between the years 2020 and 2030. Although the WHO considers health a multifaceted term, controversy and confusion still exist about whether the best health status is mandatory to age better. Because the concept of health is not even universally accepted among the general population. It needs more awareness to represent health as a multidimensional entity rather than being unidirectional. For example, why do we not age better with blooming relationships even after having some comorbidities? The term "healthy aging" is widespread. However, how appropriate it is in the truest sense of the term? Perhaps the term "better aging" or "aging well" would be more appropriate to indicate the good aging status of an individual.

According to Dr. Laura L. Carstensen, our society needs to find creative ways to use maximally our older generations, their experience and their wisdom (Carstensen, 2014). To date, aging is considered a negative part of the human life course, and different media portrayals are conveying this message to a more significant portion of society. This attitude is more prominent in Western culture than in its Eastern counterpart. However, with the change of life span development and masking the physical and mental changes that usually come with age progression, the old concepts change gradually and show that aging has an upside. Now we have realized that the fast-growing older adult population has so much potency to contribute to society, and we should use this as a growing resource in the coming days. Now we have learned that this is not a short-term effect of the baby boomers' aging, but the changing pattern of aging is going to persist for a long time, and it will be wise for us to use this significant resource. Therefore, we need to change our focus away from the negativity and inabilities associated with older age. Instead, we should rethink the potentiality of the aging mind and consider our older generation as the wiser generation, because the deterioration of one's physical health only does not mean that everything is lost. Alternatively, we should think that as people grow old, they develop some strategies from their learning processes in their life course, which help them to compensate and overcome burdens. So, they approach any problem differently than their younger counterparts because they have already experienced the youth in their life course. However, younger generations do not have the advantage of being old.

This change in individuals' realization is not specific to a particular geographical location. Thanks to modern medical technologies, public health promotions, agricultural reforms, and a multidirectional educational system, we are moving forward in every part of the globe. The modern aging society is also a result of these reforms. As members of the contemporary generation, many of us have firsthand experience that it is the "willpower" that is needed most for anyone to achieve success. When a person does (or achieves) something that is not usual for that age (or community or standard), we designate the activity as "rare" or "exceptional." However, when this happens repeatedly and by many others of that age (or community or standard), it no longer remains an exception. It is considered usual, and gradually that becomes a societal norm or government policy. The age of retirement is showing an increasing trend in different countries gradually. We are feeling the necessity of using these experienced brains, at least in some professions. Therefore, consciously or unconsciously, we are accepting the use of these elderly resources. This trend is not right in some situations, especially if we consider some overpopulated countries like India, where unemployment is a big issue. However, we should also create alternative ways for the younger generation but should not stop reusing those experienced resources. If we follow the present regulations only, we cannot move forward; instead, we should have an optimistic attitude toward making our society wealthier and more productive.

Growing old is not an easy achievement, both on bodies and minds. "Anyone can be young; it takes talent to be old!" (Poo, 2016, p.30). Greater longevity is considered a big public health victory; however, not every older adult is experiencing the equal advantage of this resource. We need to explore various creative ways so that we can use our older generation's brains maximally. Work does not mean only physical strain; it is synonymous with meaningful engagement, which could be achieved through educational engagement, cultural engagement, or productive engagement. Therefore, we need to find innovative ideas to engage our older adults with our societies. On the one hand, this complementary relationship will strengthen intergenerational bonding; on the other hand, it will contribute some beneficial effects in their longevity because accumulating evidence suggests that social and productive engagements are beneficial for longevity (Menec, 2003). In this context, in India, since it became independent from British rule in 1947, a reservation/quota system persists for the minority group, comprising some religions, castes, and women, but how long will we continue this demarcation only based on sex, ethnicity, and religion? Now, it is the time to raise our voice against the current system and preserve the term (and benefits of) "reservation" only for the older adult population. We should use their brain and expertise only, not their physical strength, after their traditional retirement. The age limit, whether it is lifelong or until they wish to work, may vary from country to country, but the idea should be the same. Another thing we should keep in mind is to take adequate measures on population control. Only announcements of one- or two-child norms would not solve anything; instead, it should be followed up strictly, and that is only possible under strict monitoring from government setup. However, if we use the government platform only for politics (in other words, "vote/election politics") and take no measure on birth control, we cannot accommodate our people in the near future. The result will not be a positive one from a global perspective, as well.

There is a black cloud that prevails in the form of late-life depression, affecting the so-called rehabilitation program of our elderly population. In the article, "Depression in the Elderly," Dr. George S. Alexopoulos discussed the present scenario of depression among older adults and future remedies from a physician's point of view. Though the data in his study are based on the elderly population of the United States, the problem is a global one. The article is very significant in the present day, and the discussion was a very in-depth one. Late-life depression usually arises in the 65+-year age group, and in most cases, it is accompanied by some chronic medical illness and cognitive impairment (Alexopoulos, 2005). Though late-life depression has some hereditary predisposing factors, institutional medical therapy (for some other diseases) is also a common factor associated with this (Alexopoulos, 2005). As the therapeutic outcome is not so productive to date, we must build positive mental health from today onward to fight against late-life depression, and the awareness should be started from early life. Education has a significant influence on late-life depression and the so-called rehabilitation program for older adults. We must engage them even after formal retirement, at least in family life, so that they never feel lonely; once there is stagnation in lifestyle, mental health is adversely affected. This engagement is also a way to achieve healthy and successful aging.

Successful aging is not a simple concept to define. It has been a long-standing debate in gerontology for many decades. Individuals' expectations in life, their coping styles, economic strain, as well as lifestyle patterns such as social interactions, culture, and genetic patterns shape one's personality and have a crucial impact on the enormous complexities of individuals' successful aging. Many scholars explored the idea of successful aging from different perspectives. Erikson's concept (1950) is considered one of the oldest thoughts on successful aging. Erikson described eight stages of the human life span covering the period of infancy to old age, in which he presented the seventh and eighth stages as adulthood and old age. "Havighurst's proposition" (1963), on the other hand, was a discussion of two contrasting theories of successful aging, namely, activity theory and disengagement theory (Martin et al., 2015). Baltes and Baltes (1990) depicted successful aging as one's development across the life course through an intertwined process of three components: selection, optimization, and compensation. Fries's (1990) discussion was focused on the compression of morbidity in the later years of life. Kahana and Kahana (1996) presented their stress-theory-based conceptual model; they highlighted self-evaluation of success, life satisfaction, meaning in life, and valued activities as most important (Martin et al., 2015). Tornstam (2005) introduced the concept of gerotranscendence in his developmental theory. However, probably the most prominent and widely accepted model of successful aging was proposed by Rowe and Kahn (1997), which encompasses freedom from disease and disability, high cognitive and physical functioning, and active engagement with life. Increased social engagement has a beneficial effect on cognitive functioning among older adults. Physical activity undoubtedly increases cognitive functioning among older adults. Also, preserved cognitive functioning is essential in older adults to remain active and healthy. This helps older adults lead an independent lifestyle and stay socially involved, thus acting as a factor to overcome loneliness, boredom, and helplessness. These, in turn, help them to remain engaged with life. Although challenging, even with deteriorating physical and cognitive health, one can still maintain their active engagement with life because of their acceptance in the family or society. Therefore, active engagement with life is probably the most vital component of successful aging.

Another prominent model that described successful aging in older adults with its analytical framework is the Baltes and Baltes selection, optimization, and compensation (SOC) model (Baltes & Baltes, 1990). As a developmental model, the SOC model explains several common human behaviors that are used to achieve the highest beneficial result through adaptation. This model supports recognizing the behavioral, motivational, and cognitive processes associated with successful aging. Accumulating evidence suggests that increased social engagement is beneficial for better cognitive functioning among older adults (Baltes & Baltes, 1990). Physical activity undoubtedly increases cognitive performance among older adults. Furthermore, preserved cognitive functioning is considered crucial for older adults to maintain an active and healthy life. This helps older adults lead an independent lifestyle, which supports them to stay socially involved and acts as a factor to overcome three classical plagues, i.e., loneliness, boredom, and helplessness. Baltes and Baltes did not shy away from discussing the losses of aging but showed some optimism regarding how losses not only can be attenuated but that aging can bring unique positive benefits such as wisdom as well.

On the other hand, Depp and Jeste (2006) emphasized a biopsychosocial definition, which should be more acceptable to clinicians, researchers, and older adults (Martin et al., 2015). In one study, Depp and Jeste (2006) reported that they found 29 definitions of successful aging; however, the most comprehensive definition should also incorporate biopsychosocial measures instead of just biomedical ones (Carr & Weir, 2017; Jeste et al., 2010). While defining successful aging, most Western researchers' definition describes freedom from disease and disability (Jeste et al., 2010); on the other hand, non-Western literature mostly focuses on adaptation, meaningfulness, connection, acknowledgment, and spirituality (Amin, 2017; Hilton et al., 2012; Lamb, 2014). Previous studies found successful aging to be influenced by many factors, such as marital status, workability, practicing healthy activities, social interaction, and strong religious beliefs (Pruchno et al., 2010). These findings are highlighted when researchers analyzed successful aging from older adults' perspectives (Amin, 2017; Phelan et al., 2004). However, Jeste et al. (2010) classified successful aging into two fundamental types: objective and subjective. They delineated the objective concept as measurable physical and mental characteristics and the subjective one as the adaptation within society and meaningfulness of life. It seems from the earlier studies, the conception of successful aging is more closely aligned with the subjective perception of an individual than objective measurement, especially at the later ages (Jeste et al., 2010; Lamb, 2014; Vaillant, 2002). Objective components are relatively easy to measure; however, subjective components are not. Subjective assessments mostly depend on the personality and psychological adaptability and resilience of the concerned individual. A substantial amount of research was carried out in the past years focusing on the determinants and application of successful aging. However, a long-standing debate on successful aging on the components and conceptualization of successful aging also continues in parallel. For instance, Rowe and Kahn's (1997) model could not provide enough explanation about subjective perceptions of well-being or meaning of life as determinants (Aldwin et al., 2006). The model only focused on late adulthood as a static assessment of an individual's successful aging. Their model did not address social structure; moreover, even though their suggested model included three essential components for optimal aging, the focus of their model did not include developmental perspectives on aging (Cho et al., 2015). Therefore, to address any discrepancies regarding the assessment of successful aging, subjective perception should be considered as more important than objective measurement. Successful aging is a relative term and shows great inter- and intraindividual variances, thus always important from the person's perspective. In other words, successful aging appears to be a multidimensional concept to guide individuals to age well; it is an accomplishment, which is mostly reflected in one's quality of life and is best justified by including subjective measures (Martin & Poon, 2016; Shrira et al., 2019).

However, successful aging is not just a box where we can input older adults with an expectation that after 20 or 30 years, they will result in survivors, delayers, or escapers (this is a categorization of 80+-year-old adults based on their health status). Older adults are not machinery products, and successful aging cannot be achieved through any mechanical (or theoretical) way. There must be some fundamental difference between success, that is, the accomplishment of goals, and satisfaction, that is, the fulfillment of expectations. The former is mostly judged by others, while the latter is typically self-centered. Self-satisfaction can be achieved professionally, through spirituality or by other means. However, one thing that impacts both success and satisfaction, which most researchers forgot to consider, is "acceptance," accepted by others at any level, and this acceptance must come with pleasure, not through any obligation or fear. Social acceptance and active engagement are interrelated and positively affect each other. Although they differ at the individual (e.g., sociodemographic parameters, interpersonal relationships) and societal (e.g., government policy) levels, they show substantial difference at family and society levels because in some cultures, the family possesses a responsibility with a strong intergenerational bonding that differs from a societal perspective. Therefore, the term successful aging cannot be restricted to some mere theoretical knowledge. As health is a combination of physical, mental, environmental, social, and spiritual factors, successful aging posits a strong connection with well-being, society, spirituality, and wisdom. *Bhagavad Gita*, one of the most venerated philosophical texts in Hinduism, guides us about a range of wisdom, where the ancient yogis were ranked at the highest level. They accomplished their success through arduous meditation and subsequent achievement of wisdom. This concept of successful aging is still significant in the present world. A few examples are Mahatma Gandhi, George Bernard Shaw, Mother Teresa, and Nelson Mandela, international role models who were accepted at much broader levels, but anyone can achieve this success even at the family or community levels. This acceptance brings joyous feelings to the person that cannot be limited by counting only the number of a few extra years in later life. For instance, if a person dies between 65 and 70 years after leading a blissful and accepted life without having any morbidity, is that considered to be unsuccessful aging? Perhaps the term "successful aging" makes our thought process more unidirectional. "Joyful aging" would be a much better term to indicate aging successfully.

I know one gentleman personally, Mr. Barun Kumar Bhattacharya, who is 75 years old but has a fit body both physically and mentally. He is a chartered accountant by profession and a regular trekker by passion. A few months back, he did a successful summit trek of 21,000 feet without an oxygen cylinder. He is self-dependent, lives with his spouse, and looks younger than his chronological age. He only came to my clinic to check his blood pressure regularly but never was sick. In my eyes, his self-motivating lifestyle is a typical example of successful aging, i.e., uplifting the human body physically and psychologically fit over its chronological age. Therefore, we can conclude that "better aging" or "aging well" is possible in every part of this world, not only in a particular country, but proper planning is necessary, whether the motivation comes from the individual, the society, or the government.

4.2 Determinants of Aging Well

4.2.1 Personality

Personality is commonly defined as the individual differences between people in their patterns of thinking, feeling, and behaving. This is an important contributor to an individual's mental health. However, there is no consensus on the timing of initiation and extent of cognitive decline. Some researchers argue that the beginning of cognitive decline starts as early as the 20s, while others suggest this decline in cognitive functioning begins during the middle ages or even later. Whatever may be the timing and extent of cognitive decline, progressive deterioration of cognitive function can lead to further cognitive impairment and dementia. Research has widely documented that personality is associated with cognitive decline in older ages, thus having an impact on individuals' health (Sadeq & Molinari, 2018). The basic aspects of cognition, such as memory, attention, and processing speed, show a gradual decline with age, even though intraindividual variability influences the cognitive performance of older adults. Research also suggests that personality change in adulthood is related to physical health and longevity (Graham & Lachman, 2012).

According to the previous studies, an intimate relationship exists between personality variables like traits and motives with the health status of an individual. Both wellness and illness could lead one to live a restructured life by changing their personality and vice versa. The big five personality traits that were identified are extraversion, agreeableness, conscientiousness, neuroticism, and openness (McCrae & Costa, 1987). These influence an individual's health outcome (Hill & Roberts, 2016). Many studies suggested personality characteristics as possible predictors of some of the intraindividual variability in cognitive aging. Trait theories of cognition describe the way people differ from one another in their stable behavioral patterns. Personality traits (such as openness and conscientiousness) and interests (particularly those that are realistic) together determine the intensity and direction of one's intellectual investment. The cumulative investment of intellectual effort is suggested to have an impact on the development of intelligence depending on individual choices (Graham & Lachman, 2012). For example, individuals more inclined toward neuroticism have been proven to be anxious and vulnerable to stress, thereby remembering fewer words, while conscientiousness tends to be associated with better performance on a range of tasks due to better cognitive health. On the other hand, the social-cognitive perspective on personality theory describes various cognitive processes, such as thinking and judging, affecting the development of an individual's personality. These cognitive processes influence the learned behaviors that build one's personality. These learned behaviors have a big impact linking personality traits to cognition in old age. According to some scholars, personality processes are means that ultimately flourish to yield the effects of personality traits (Hampson, 2012). Although controversies still exist on the exact mechanism that links personality traits to cognition in old age, the cumulative investment of intellectual effort along with the learned behaviors is the most important mechanism that correlates personality traits with cognition in late life.

Disengagement theory suggests that older adults purposely withdraw from society. This is particularly important when older adults retire from work and decrease their social participation. On the contrary, activity theory suggests that healthy aging (or aging well) corresponds with continued psychological engagement and social participation throughout older age. Thus, older adults should actively compensate for the age-related changes in their mental, biological, and social experiences, and individuals must continue to be involved in meaningful activities as health promotion measures. Neuroticism is probably the most common personality trait examined in conjunction with negative health behavior. It is characterized by negative emotions, such as anger, anxiety, and depression; it has been suggested to be a risk factor for increasing stress levels. On the other hand, conscientiousness is arguably the personality trait most likely to be implicated in health-promoting behavior and social engagement. Thus, in my opinion, personality trait is directly related to both physical and mental health in older adults.

According to Kandler et al. (2015), change in perceived control was associated with alterations in neuroticism and conscientiousness, signifying the relation of some specific adaptation to old age. They concluded that individual well-being decreases with strongly increasing levels of neuroticism and decreasing extraversion, conscientiousness, and perceived control, suggesting personality traits impact well-being but not vice versa. On the other hand, studying 5,200 older adults over a span of 4 years, Stephan et al. (2016) found that physiological dysregulation across multiple systems challenges personality stability and may even alter accelerated personality traits. It has been found that personality tends to get better over time. Psychologists consider this as "the maturity principle" (Van den Akker et al., 2014). People become more extraverted, emotionally stable, agreeable, and conscientious as they grow older. Life events, like marriage and childbirth, help them to change over time.

Furthermore, some strong interrelationships exist between personality traits and different biological markers of the aging process and health; for instance, conscientious and less neurotic individuals tend to exhibit reduced interleukin-6 (IL-6). Conscientiousness has been proven to be an influential factor that protects against Alzheimer's disease (Hill & Roberts, 2016). Usually, older adults show less neurotic behavior than their younger counterparts regarding alcohol and tobacco use, risky driving, unhealthy dietary habits, and mental activity. Also, different biomarkers play roles of varying intensity in different periods of life. A strong interrelationship exists between longevity and different personality traits. Centenarians usually have "low neuroticism, high conscientiousness and moderate levels of extraversion and agreeableness" (Smith & Ryan, 2016, p. 309). Self-related belief is also an influential factor here because it may show thankfulness to everyone for having lived for such a long time. Still, they also fear and worry about their declining physical and mental health. They often show reluctance to make the future for the rest of life and gradually become pessimistic in attitude, mainly due to their social losses, as their social connections usually start declining over time (Smith & Ryan, 2016). For this reason, social isolation and connections are strongly related to increased mortality and morbidity risks.

At this point of discussion, I want to mention one of my patients, who is substantially related to the current topic. The person was a merchant navy officer before retirement and enjoyed his life in an undisciplined manner. He had different addictions and uncontrolled dietary habits until his mid-60s when he experienced a life-changing medical event (stroke); as a consequence, one side of his body was paralyzed (hemiplegia). He was very upset at that time, but he always possessed an optimistic attitude in his life. So, after his recovery, he started to lead an almost austere lifestyle with a vegetarian diet, yoga (with physical exercise and meditation), and an introverted appearance, which redirected him toward a conscientious path. We were very much surprised as we have never seen him before with that personality. Now he is in his early 80s, and, according to him, he is enjoying life in a better way.

4.2.2   Interpersonal Relationships

Another crucial determinant of "better aging" is the positive relationship between married couples. Levels of the well-being of spouses are intimately related to each other and help the couple to attain better aging together. Although biologically unrelated to each other, spouses usually spend a considerable and vital time of their life span with each other in the same environment. As a consequence, they recognize the positive and negative aspects of their partners and compensate each other during their substantial period of coexistence (Hoppmann & Gerstorf, 2016). This compensation and optimization have a significant impact on their aging outcomes, even during their individual losses, from the perspective of leading an optimal quality of life with minimal health hazards (Hoppmann & Gerstorf, 2016). A positive psychological bonding develops in the spousal relationship that has a beneficial impact in their age-related morbidities, including cognitive decline, even mortality. Research has found that a good marriage at 50 years predicts positive aging at 80 years (Vaillant, 2002). In contrast, a negative atmosphere in a spousal relationship elevates chances of stress and thereby related morbidities. By virtue of their close companionship for a longer period, older spouses usually show more intimacy with fewer conflicts compared to their younger counterparts, to maintain this social relationship (Fingerman & Charles, 2010). It has been found that older couples are treated with more respect and dignity by their social companions, possibly because of their experiences and kind management abilities (Fingerman & Charles, 2010). As time progresses, a spousal relationship usually turns into a feeling of commitment due to the responsibility and caring for each other (Kemp, 2008). It has already been established that happy marital relationship has benefits to maintain physical and mental health in many ways (Umberson et al., 2013). These protective health benefits are found to be greater in the spousal relationship than in any other social relation (Kim & McKenry, 2002; Stanton, 2012).

In Indian culture, organized social marriage is still considered an unofficial norm and considered the biggest event in life (Sharma et al., 2013). Religious faith, family tradition, and overall sociocultural values significantly impact marital arrangements and sustain marital relations in India (Bowman & Dollahite, 2013). Many consider this relation a sacred one, a God's directive set even before their birth. Many others are not so devoted; however, they continue the relationship for social acceptability, as if a porcupine and a rabbit were residing in the same cage, and even under a crisis that impacts the stability of marriage, social values protect against catastrophes (Singh, 2010). Though the newer generation is coming out of this norm, they prefer to select their life partners independently, and the number of those living together shows an increasing trend. Still, the divorce rate is much less (1%) than in many other countries, probably because, in most cases, marital relationship is viewed with respect and considered as the most personal relationship. However, not only the marital relationship, but also close companionship in any relationship has been proven to have a beneficial effect on aging that is better for an individual. In India, extended multigenerational family culture is a social norm, and it plays a significant role in longevity and aging well through emotional bonding and discipline.

However, some variations exist in relationships between older adults in a European-American culture based on negative stereotypes. Therefore, I was surprised when I first met the couple, Amy and Kenneth Knoespel (my new friends in the United States), who have already celebrated their 50th wedding anniversary in 2018. They have strong social connections. Amy is doing her master's degree in gerontology in her early 70s and is still eager to do something for society, especially for the older adults, and at the same time, she wants to prove herself.

4.3   Challenges of Aging Well

The aging of the population has a profound influence on the lives of individuals everywhere. The success of people's material and psychological well-being depends on the policies taken by the concerned government on health and healthcare, education, work and retirement, and family life sectors. Toni Antonucci and colleagues have shown in their article that although present-day America is a few steps ahead of other countries in many respects in the domain of aging, it still is not fully prepared in front of the new challenges of demographic revolution (Antonucci et al., 2016). We are passing through a time when the "third demographic dividend" for aging societies is due. We are at a time juncture when our society is facing challenges with a sudden increase in the number of older adults in with very little opportunity and caregivers for them. Therefore, the psychological well-being of individuals largely depends on multidisciplinary collaborations. To achieve that psychological well-being, one of the essential parameters is education, which, according to the author, affects the entire course of life. They are intimately interconnected, particularly at a time when family structure is changing. A good and pragmatic education is necessary to achieve a healthy life, and in this regard, the young-old generation is having more education than their parents' generation. Obviously, they are more fit than their parents were at the same age point. For this reason, they are excellent resources for society, as they can be engaged either through paid work or volunteering, which is beneficial for both them and their society. Economic security is the most concerning factor after retirement, and this cannot be achieved without having a healthy life. The most challenging part of the present-day United States is to provide healthcare costs. With this perspective, both work and family life are significant. Healthcare cost is a tremendous burden, whether it is long-term or short-term care. Especially where long-term care is required, the concerned family faces a huge economic challenge. Whether informal care is needed, for which one or more family members become(s) engaged and unavailable to others (even for their own requirement), or formal care is required, the cost of which, the concerned family cannot bear most of the time. Above all, when the concerned older adult is alone or in a nuclear family, the burden becomes multiple. During my higher studies in the United States, I met Mr. Neil Fleming, who later became our family friend. Neil is a divorced gentleman in his early 70s who lives alone in his condominium. He is very enthusiastic, a cyclist by passion, and self-motivated to complete his master's degree in gerontology with an eagerness to do something beneficial for the older adult community.

In India, the government incorporated an act for the care and protection of older adults by their children. "The Maintenance and Welfare of Parents and Senior Citizen Act, 2007" was enacted to benefit the elderly people; some policy like that is necessary in the United States as well. However, for a successful implementation, proper follow-up of those policies is also essential. While doing that, the government also has a responsibility to assure the work-life balance of the so-called sandwich generation; otherwise, after a couple of decades, we will be in a questionable situation again.

Therefore, the long-standing debate still exists on reaching a consensus on the ideas of "better aging" and its nourishment. We have discussed normal psychological aging and mental health, "joyful" aging, and the most common types of behavioral health problems, encircling the main point that aging is not a disease. Our intention to define aging attempts to label people in yet another way and put them in groups in a highly subjective manner. By definition, pathology is the medical domain that deals with conditions typically observed during a disease state. In contrast, physiology is the biological domain that describes processes or mechanisms operating normally within an organism. I am often confused that we do not consider the medical discipline as a biological one. When our cardiac cells deteriorate in their function, it is pathology, but when our brain cells show a decline in function, it is physiology. How? Why is there not a universal age of cognitive decline that is considered due to aging? Why are we concerned about preventing cognitive degeneration as we age if it is a normal physiology? We discuss a lot about adjustment issues in later life that may lead to adjustment disorders. It could be a late-life manifestation, but does it originate only in later life? Doesn't it start from the day we come out of our mother's womb? Or perhaps even earlier than that? Various models/theories in gerontology guide us on successful aging, but what is the age range that this guidance covers? Does any model tell us anything on how to nurture a toddler to achieve a so-called successful aging? Indeed, we are concentrating so much on the terminologies that we are going far from the center of the problems. Our primary purpose is to extract something for ourselves from this subject. We do not think beyond our territories. For instance, now, in my mid-40s, I often forget about many daily activities that I could not imagine forgetting at least 10 years ago. Is it physiology or pathology? Who will judge this? Which medical professional? Everyone is different. Everyone's life course is different. Everyone's life stressors are different, different even much more than their thumbprint variations.

At this point of discussion, an obvious question arises: who is responsible for all these happenings? Are we not making our future more complicated? To find the answer, we must explore the history of geropsychology. Birren and Schroots, in their book chapter "The History of Geropsychology" (Birren & Schroots, 2001), presented a detailed argument that human aging is the result of ecological relationships. They have argued that since the time of mythological origin, i.e., sometime around 3000 BC through subsequent periods, aging was defined from multiple perspectives. There were some beliefs that many people attained excess longevity in that ancient time; however, there was no such positive approach regarding aging well. It was Plato who first emphasized that "to age wisely and peacefully, it is necessary to live a righteous life" (Birren & Schroots, 2001; p.7), and to achieve this, education with a sense of responsibility is needed from younger life. This education is exactly what we are discussing regarding the present day's view on aging. However, the authors only addressed the Western literature records. Perhaps the current discussion will remain incomplete if we do not compare this notion with non-Western literature. In India, in one of the ancient sets of literature of human civilization, the Upanishads, around the seventh to sixth centuries BCE (King, 1995; although Stephen Phillips chronologized the oldest Upanishads in the 800 to 300 BCE range [Philips, 2009]), four stages were mentioned in the human life course. Each was called an "ashram": first, "Brahmacharya" (the period of learning/studentship); second, "Garhasthya" (the period of family life); third, "Vanaprastha" (the period when one hands over the household duties to their successors and becomes free from family responsibilities); and finally, "Sanyas" (the period when one starts leading an utterly secluded life, free of worldly things). Since the Vedic period, these stages were considered to create and sustain a social discipline, peace, and harmony (Tiwary & Pandey, 2013). Each of these stages was limited to roughly 25 years. Therefore, it can be assumed that many centenarians achieved these stages even during the Vedic period (Bhattacharyya, 2017), although this achievement requires discipline, bonding, and sacrifices as well. Therefore, proper education and a disciplined lifestyle are necessary to achieve "better aging," i.e., "aging well." It can also be stated from the opposite perspective that aging will be better if the older adults sacrifice properly in their later years; the expectation of a huge outcome from later life is not wise.

4.4 Conclusion

In recent years, the World Health Organization has initiated a campaign to create and sustain age-friendly communities across the world (World Health Organization, 2007a, b). Aging is a lifelong process. Therefore, age-friendly communities are not only aiming to be "older adult-friendly"; instead, this movement also is structured on eight priority domains that target creating active aging communities that engage every older adult at all life stages and abilities. Those eight priority sectors include housing, transportation, social participation, respect and social inclusion, civic participation and employment, communication and information, community support and health services, and outdoor spaces and buildings (De Biasi et al., 2020). An ideal age-friendly community should be accessible, equitable, inclusive, safe, secure, and supportive (World Health Organization, 2007a, b). However, in a country with a vast population, where distinct demarcation exists in culture, language, and economic status, the concept of a segregated but happy older adult community seems impractical, at least without a distinct social stratification. Age-friendly communities may start at home; it is not only about changing the outer world but also changing our minds. An age-friendly community is possible only within the general population, within a multigenerational environment. Currently, the "aging in place" movement is showing a growing trend as a cost-effective measure for individuals who can stay longer at home instead of at an institution. Millions of older adults want to "age in place." They want to stay in their home environment, safely and independently, wishing to avoid staying in an age-segregated community, far away from their hometown. We are making our life complex and then finding a way out. Following the traditional route of lifestyle, we can find the significance of aging in place and an age-friendly community.

References

Aldwin, C. M., Spiro, A., III, & Park, C. L. (2006). Health, behavior, and optimal aging: A life span developmental perspective. In J. E. Birren & K. W. Schaire (Eds.), *Handbook of the psychology of aging* (pp. 85–104). Elsevier. https://doi.org/10.1016/B978-012101264-9/50008-2

Alexopoulos, G. S. (2005). Depression in the elderly. *Lancet, 365*, 1961–1970.

Amin, I. (2017). Perceptions of successful aging among older adults in Bangladesh: An exploratory study. *Journal of Cross-Cultural Gerontology, 32*(2), 191–207. https://doi.org/10.1007/s10823-017-9319-3

Antonucci, T. C., Berkman, L., Borsch-Supan, A., Carstense, L. L., Fried, L. P., Furstenberg, F. F., Goldman, D., Jackson, J. S., Kohli, M., Olshansky, S. J., Rother, J., Rowe, J. W., & Zissimopoulos, J. (2016). Society and the individual at the dawn of the twenty-first century. In K. W. Schaie & S. L. Willis (Eds.), *Handbook of psychology of aging* (8th ed., pp. 42–58). Academic Press.

Baltes, P. B., & Baltes, M. M. (1990). Psychological perspectives on successful aging: The model of selective optimization with compensation. In P. B. Baltes P. B., & M. M. Baltes (Eds.), *Successful aging: Perspectives from the behavioral sciences* (pp. 1–34). United Kingdom: Cambridge University Press.

Bhattacharyya, K. K. (2017). Centenarians in India: The present scenario. *International Journal of Community Medicine and Public Health, 4*(7), 2219–2225. https://doi.org/10.18203/2394-6040.ijcmph20172809

Birren, J. E., & Schroots, J. J. F. (2001). The history of geropsychology. In K. W. Schaie & S. L. Willis (Eds.), *Handbook of the psychology of aging* (6th ed., pp. 3–26). Academic Press.

Bowman, J., & Dollahite, D. (2013). "Why would such a person dream about heaven?" Family, faith, and happiness in arranged marriages in India. *Journal of Comparative Family Studies, 44*(2), 207–225.

Carr, K., & Weir, P. L. (2017). A qualitative description of successful aging through different decades of older adulthood. *Aging & Mental Health, 21*(12), 1317–1325. https://doi.org/10.1080/13607863.2016.1226764

Carstensen, L. L. (2014). Our aging population—it may save us all. In P. H. Irving (Ed.), *The upside of aging: How long life is changing the world of health, work, innovation, policy, and purpose*. Wiley.

Cho, J., Martin, P., Poon, L. W., & Georgia Centenarian Study. (2015). Successful aging and subjective well-being among oldest-old adults. *The Gerontologist, 55*(1), 132–143. https://doi.org/10.1093/geront/gnu074

De Biasi, A., Wolfe, M., Carmody, J., Fulmer, T., & Auerbach, J. (2020). Creating an age-friendly public health system. *Innovation in Aging, 4*(1), igz044. https://doi.org/10.1093/geroni/igz044

Fingerman, K. L., & Charles, S. T. (2010). It takes two to tango: Why older people have the best relationships. *Current Directions in Psychological Science, 19*, 172–176.

Fried, L. P. (2016). Investing in health to create a third demographic dividend. *The Gerontologist, 56*(S2), S167–S177. https://doi.org/10.1093/geront/gnw035

Graham, E. K., & Lachman, M. E. (2012). Personality stability is associated with better cognitive performance in adulthood: Are the stable more able? *The Journals of Gerontology. Series B, Psychological Sciences and Social Sciences, 67*(5), 545–554. https://doi.org/10.1093/geronb/gbr149

Hampson, S. E. (2012). Personality processes: mechanisms by which personality traits "get outside the skin". *Annual Review of Psychology, 63*, 315–339. https://doi.org/10.1146/annurev-psych-120710-100419

Hill, P. L., & Roberts, B. W. (2016). Personality and Health: Reviewing recent research and setting a directive for the future. In K. W. Schaie & S. L. Willis (Eds.), *Handbook of the psychology of aging* (8th ed., pp. 206–216). Academic Press.

Hilton, J., Gonzalez, C., Saleh, M., Maitoza, R., & Anngela-Cole, L. (2012). Perceptions of successful aging among older Latinos in cross-cultural context. *Journal of Cross-Cultural Gerontology, 27*(3), 183–199. https://doi.org/10.1007/s10823-012-9171-4

Hoppmann, C. A., & Gerstorf, D. (2016). Social interrelations in aging: The sample case of married couples. In K. W. Schaie & S. L. Willis (Eds.), *Handbook of the psychology of aging* (8th ed., pp. 263–277). Academic Press.

Jeste, D. V., Depp, C. A., & Vahia, I. V. (2010). Successful cognitive and emotional aging. *World Psychiatry, 9*(2), 78–84.

Kahana, E., & Kahana, B. (1996). Conceptual and empirical advances in understanding aging well through proactive adaptation. In V. Bengtson (Ed.), Adulthood and aging: Research on continuities and discontinuities (pp. 18–40). New York: Springer.

Kandler, C., Kornadt, A. E., Hagemeyer, B., & Neyer, F. J. (2015). Patterns and sources of personality development in old age. *Journal of Personality and Social Psychology, 109*(1), 175–191. https://doi.org/10.1037/pspp0000028

Kemp, C. L. (2008). Negotiating transitions in later life: Married couples in assisted living. *Journal of Applied Gerontology, 27*(3), 231–251.

Kim, H. K., & McKenry, P. C. (2002). The relationship between marriage and psychological well-being: A longitudinal analysis. *Journal of Family Issues, 23*, 905.

King, R. (1995). *Early Advaita Vedānta and Buddhism: The Mahāyāna context of the Gauḍapādīya-kārikā, Gauḍapāda*. State University of New York Press. ISBN 978-0-7914-2513-8.

Lamb, S. (2014). Permanent personhood or meaningful decline? Toward a critical anthropology of successful aging. *Journal of Aging Studies, 29*, 41–52. https://doi.org/10.1016/j.jaging.2013.12.006

Martin, P., & Poon, L. W. (2016). Success at 100 is easier said than done – comments on Araújo et al: Successful aging at 100 years. *International Psychogeriatrics, 28*(2), 177–178. https://doi.org/10.1017/S1041610215002021

Martin, P., Kelly, N., Kahana, B., Kahana, E., Willcox, B. J., Willcox, D. C., & Poon, L. W. (2015). Defining successful aging: A tangible or elusive concept? *The Gerontologist, 55*(1), 14–25.

McCrae, R. R., & Costa, P. T. (1987). Validation of the five-factor model of personality across instruments and observers. *Journal of Personality and Social Psychology, 52*(1), 81–90. https://doi.org/10.1037/0022-3514.52.1.81

Menec, V. H. (2003). The relation between everyday activities and successful aging: A 6-year longitudinal study. *The Journals of Gerontology. Series B, Psychological Sciences and Social Sciences, 58*(2), S74–S82. https://doi.org/10.1093/geronb/58.2.s74

Phelan, E. A., Anderson, L. A., LaCroix, A. Z., & Larson, E. B. (2004). Older adults' views of "successful aging" – How do they compare with researchers' definitions? *Journal of the American Geriatrics Society, 52*(2), 211–216. https://doi.org/10.1111/j.1532-5415.2004.52056.x

Phillips, S. H. (2009). *Yoga, karma, and rebirth: A brief history and philosophy*. Columbia University Press. ISBN 978-0231144858.

Poo, A. (2016). *The age of dignity: Preparing for the elder boom in a changing America*. The New Press.

Pruchno, R. A., Wilson-Genderson, M., Rose, M., & Cartwright, F. (2010). Successful aging: Early influences and contemporary characteristics. *The Gerontologist, 50*(6), 821–833. https://doi.org/10.1093/geront/gnq041

Rowe, J. W., & Kahn, R. L. (1997). Successful aging. *The Gerontologist, 37*(4), 433–440.

Sadeq, N. A., & Molinari, V. (2018). Personality and its relationship to depression and cognition in older adults: Implications for practice. *Clinical Gerontologist, 41*(5), 385–398. https://doi.org/10.1080/07317115.2017.1407981

Sharma, I., Pandit, B., Pathak, A., & Sharma, R. (2013). Hinduism, marriage and mental illness. *Indian Journal of Psychiatry, 55*(Suppl 2), S243–S249.

Shrira, A., Carmel, S., Tovel, H., & Raveis, V. H. (2019). Reciprocal relationships between the will-to-live and successful aging. *Aging & Mental Health, 23*(10), 1350–1357. https://doi.org/10.1080/13607863.2018.1499011

Singh, J. P. (2010). *Problems of India's changing family and state intervention*. Retrieved on July 24, 2020, from: http://www.un.org/esa/socdev/family/docs/egm09/Singh.pdf

Singh, A., & Misra, N. (2009). Loneliness, depression and sociability in old age. *Industrial Psychiatry Journal, 18*(1), 51–55. https://doi.org/10.4103/0972-6748.57861

Smith, J., & Ryan, L. H. (2016). Psychological vitality in the oldest old. In K. W. Schaie & S. L. Willis (Eds.), *Handbook of the psychology of aging* (8th ed., pp. 303–316). Academic Press.

Stanton, G. (2012). *The health benefits of marriage*. Focus on the Family. Internet source. Retrieved from: https://www.focusonthefamily.com/about/focus.../marriage/health-benefits-of-marriag

Stephan, Y., Sutin, A. R., Luchetti, M., & Terracciano, A. (2016). Allostatic load and personality: A 4-year longitudinal study. *Psychosomatic Medicine, 78*(3), 302–310. https://doi.org/10.1097/PSY.0000000000000281

Tiwari, S. C., & Pandey, N. M. (2013). The Indian concepts of lifestyle and mental health in old age. *Indian Journal of Psychiatry, 55*(Suppl S2), 288–292.

Tornstam, L. (2005). *Gerotranscendence: A developmental theory of positive aging*. New York: Springer Publishing Company.

Umberson, D., Williams, K., & Thomeer, M. B. (2013). Family status and mental health: Recent advances and future directions. In C. S. Aneshensel & J. C. Phelan (Eds.), *Handbook of the sociology of mental health* (2nd ed., pp. 405–431). Springer Publishing.

Vaillant, G. (2002). *Aging well: Surprising guideposts to a happier life from the landmark harvard study of adult development*. Little, Brown and Company.

Van den Akker, A. L., Deković, M., Asscher, J., & Prinzie, P. (2014). Mean-level personality development across childhood and adolescence: A temporary defiance of the maturity principle and bidirectional associations with parenting. *Journal of Personality and Social Psychology, 107*(4), 736–750. https://doi.org/10.1037/a0037248

World Health Organization. (2007a). *Global age-friendly cities: A guide*. World Health Organization. Retrieved from: https://www.who.int/ageing/publications/Global_age_friendly_cities_Guide_English.pdf. Accessed November 2020.

World Health Organization. (2007b). *Age-friendly environments*. World Health Organization. Retrieved from: https://www.who.int/ageing/projects/age-friendly-environments/en/. Accessed November 2020.

World Health Organization. (2020). *Decade of healthy ageing*. World Health Organization. Retrieved from: https://www.who.int/ageing/decade-of-healthy-ageing#:~:text=What%20is%20Healthy%20Ageing%3F,they%20have%20reason%20to%20value. Accessed November 2020.

Chapter 5
Aging, Caregiving, and COVID-19

5.1 Rethinking Eldercare

One of the biggest concerns of the present day's world is eldercare—whether it is healthcare or regular care for basic activities or to provide emotional and financial care. Is this care necessary for every older adult? However, the main question is, who will care? Do the responsibilities belong to the family members only or society (or community) or country (or the government), or does the person concerned have some of their own responsibilities? When it is the concern of the family members (or the next generation), is it their sole responsibility, sacrificing their own demands? However, when the responsibilities come on the country's shoulder, then the question arises, "Which country?"—the country where the concerned person was born, raised, and worked, investing their physical and mental energies and at last expects some positive feedback? Or the country where they have migrated in later ages, even without having mental bonding with this new country? The answers are still very cloudy.

To emphasize the role of caregivers, Rosalynn Carter once shared, "There are only four kinds of people in the world: those who have been caregivers, those who are currently caregivers, those who will be caregivers, and those who will need caregivers" (Carter & Golant, 1994, p.1). In all practical reality, every long-term care experience is based on this idea, once realized by the former US first lady. The act of caregiving can be viewed from many angles. While caring for a dementia patient, the primary caregiver feels stress for the continuous monotonous duty as a caregiver; their frustration is not to leave their spouse alone even for a few minutes, despite having their own health problems. They feel stress thinking that if they suffer from any major health problem, who will take care of their partner? Other than performing basic daily activities for themselves and assisting spouses, they must arrange for meals, financial work like bank dealings, transportation, medical consultation, and social connection maintenance. These can lead the caregiver toward severe depression and increase the risk of mortality, too. In most cases, they are technologically savvy, socially isolated, and reluctant to proceed with any physical exercise program. The gap with the next generation is gradually increasing, and they feel lonely and isolated from a negative feedback effect. Traditional extended family culture has profound importance here. In Indian family culture, the daughter-in-law plays a considerable role in the eldercare segment; this is an ideal example of a feminine role in maintaining and protecting the societal structure. However, it seems, somehow, we are heading in the opposite direction.

In the book *The Age of Dignity...*, Poo (2016) has described a few characters in a vivid style so that we could feel it in a personalized manner. The author tried to picture the eldercare scenario with different lively examples and research data in present-day America. It seems she is very much successful in her intention in front of the readers. According to her, the most negative aspects in this regard are the increasing cost and shortage of dedicated caregivers in the present-day United States. Poo pointed out that the success of our current healthcare system is measured by how it delays death rather than supports the quality of life. This problem is a fundamental one anywhere in the world, whether it is a developed country or a developing one. It is obvious that everybody might not be so lucky, like Poo's grandmother, who could get assistance from generous Mrs. Sun. There may not be a caregiver like Mrs. Sun everywhere. Good care not only means providing some clinical measures to relieve the symptoms; instead, care with dignity and continuity of services is also crucial so that the concerned person feels comfortable, irrespective of whether the care is done at home or in an institutional setting. There must be some mental bonding from either side, whether the care comes from a professional or a family member.

We indeed need to rethink everything—not only how we live, work, and enjoy our own life but also how we take care of each other across generations. As members of the contemporary generation, many of us have firsthand experience as care providers. Simultaneously, we also realize that often we cannot make significant changes in their lives and cannot give them that level of satisfaction, what they want in later life, so that we need to find the way out. Even though we are not solely responsible for the care, we are unable to provide them with this care because the situation does not always permit us. Therefore, what will be the fate of our next generation of older adults? Do they spend their later life in a segregated and neglected way, in so-called old age homes? Or we can provide them a better future with home care in the later years of their life or high-quality institutional care settings when necessary. However, presently, we, the so-called sandwich generation, are also in a state of confusion. Should we take steps that also will be beneficial in our later lives, bringing experience from the mistakes of our previous generation? The current COVID-19 pandemic has further compounded the difficulties, both for caregivers and care recipients. It has become an enormous difficulty for even the long-distance caregivers to care for their loved ones during an apparently strict and confusing situation of social distancing, at the same time when we do not have any control over transportation and other basic amenities. Everyone is facing this stifling situation, but the solution is far out of sight.

Are we responsible for the effects of "the elder boom?" Are we responsible for the government policy of one- or two-child norms, which affected our parents, and that is why we do not have any (or many) siblings? Are we responsible for the then socioeconomic condition for which our parents could not save much in their retirement benefit plan? However, society's spotlight is on us—the "sandwich generation"; we are feeling guilty about those unwanted situations related to the present condition of elderly people with which we do not have any direct relation at all. This situation seems to be an apparent gap between older adults and their next generation. The persistence of this gap is a glaring fault of the government of different countries that do not have some universal policies in place related to these social problems.

The present life is so fast that economic reforms and urbanization are making people self-reliant in a busy life schedule. We found this example in an elaborated study by Dr. Zhan et al. (2006). However, the traditional filial eldercare is not possible for the sandwich generation, who remains confused in a continuous "push and pull situation" from the opposite direction (Zhan et al., 2006). In this study, the authors have discussed eldercare from a global perspective, based on Chinese healthcare systems. The article's primary intention is the same: differences are only in the presentation and location.

Therefore, who is responsible for the present situation of eldercare? Ferraro and Shippee (2009) have described the complex cumulative inequality theory in such an easily digestible way that everyone can understand its significance. According to the article, "Aging and cumulative inequality…," at least our generation, is not solely responsible for the current neglected scenario of eldercare. This theory "gives special attention to family lineage and, concomitantly, reproduction, gestation, and childhood" to create a bridge to understand origin and senescence (Ferraro & Shippee, 2009). It is a view of the link between early life origin and health in later life. The concept is very much similar to what we found in a well-known mythological story. In India, in the Hindu epic "The Mahabharata," once-lord Sri Krishna was narrating the art of breaking the *Chakrabyuha* (the netlike battle formation by seven fighters of the *Kaurava Army*) and how to win that war to Subhadra (sister of Lord Sri Krishna and wife of Arjuna). During the latter part of the story, Subhadra slept, so she could not listen to the last part of the story, i.e., how to escape the *Chakrabyuha*. Abhimanyu (son of Subhadra and Arjuna) learned the art of breaking into the *Chakrabyuha* when he was in Subhadra's womb. However, he did not know how to destroy that formation once he is inside (as his mother did not hear). While in the Kurukshetra war, the promising teenaged fighter Abhimanyu entered the powerful *Chakrabyuha*, had a hard fight but could not escape that network, and was ultimately killed by the Kaurava army. Although Abhimanyu was much younger, there might be some correlation between this story and the cumulative inequality theory. Therefore, every event in our life is somehow related to our past actions (*karma*) and follows the cumulative inequality theory. However, the cumulative inequality theory may not be an excuse for our individual responsibility; we have to look forward with a positive approach. We should respect our elderly population and their moral values and wisdom, and we should proceed forward with this hope so that we can provide our older adults with better health and quality aging.

5.2   Rethinking Kinship Care

Kinship care is another type of care approach where the care may not always be associated with the diseased condition. This is a transition in the caring role that we are discussing; here, the grandparents are raising their grandchildren. In this caring role, they have to face many difficulties in their daily lives, like poverty, housing, child education, health, and wellness. I have had some opportunities to meet some kinship caregivers in the United States, and it was very surprising to watch the bold attitude of these older adults and the way they shared their experiences and views in front of some unknown faces. Kinship services are not very popular in India; even the term itself is not very common. Although this segment of care is not uncommon in India, it is present much more in number in society and probably tackled more sensibly than it is in the United States. Many approaches are new here; still, from my standpoint, these services are not enough. Therefore, some measures may be beneficial regarding redesign of caregiver service policy. First, we must find volunteers from the informal caregivers who have firsthand experiences of caregiving in the concerned domain. They can work (their role will not be care recipient only) as a link, in collaboration with other professionals, at least at local levels. From previous experience, I realized that professionals might be biased due to factors, such as payment and popularity. However, these individuals never forget their honesty. Second, from a practical standpoint, the elderly kinship caregivers, due to their physical disability (like arthritis, cardiac problems), psychological disability (like stress and depression), and isolation (like lack of transportation), often cannot be able to provide kinship care at their best. All the programs target these people with different descriptions and goals (big theoretical sentences!); however, we should make those programs practically more feasible to get maximum outcome. Third, if we look from an international perspective, for instance, in India, there is a system called "Anganwadi." The Anganwadi workers (almost like kinship navigators) are the lowest-level health workers but have much impact on societies, especially where modern medical facilities are not readily available. They provide awareness and primary care but all in person. Therefore (especially for technologically savvy individuals), we should focus more on in-person care consultation/awareness generation instead of telephone-based care consultation. Those workers will visit the targeted population frequently. Because if someone touches a person and says, "how are you," regarding building intimacy and showing support, that is more effective than saying the same words over the telephone. Therefore, it should be our priority to establish more community centers and engage more navigators accessible to the targeted older adults in their locality. Finally, everywhere the programs are delivered through social workers, counselors, or nurses. The involvement of physicians is not significantly documented. This approach is true in every field of caregiving, as if physicians are only regarded as prescribers of medications. However, physicians can play a significant role other than this; therefore, if we design these programs in such a way that involves physicians (at least primary care physicians) actively, this will certainly increase the weight and authenticity of the programs delivered.

5.3   Long-Term Care and Nursing Homes

Long-term care usually denotes the nonmedical care provided to individuals, especially older adults, who require help to carry out the basic activities of their daily living, i.e., bathing, eating, toileting, and many others. The healthcare systems in India and the United States are distinctly different, even in the components of long-term care. In the United States, those who need specific medical attention, i.e., skilled care, usually attend hospitals. For those who do not require specific medical attention, custodial care is provided. Long-term care consists of specific services provided as informal care (e.g., by family and friends), formal care, or institutional care. Formal care may be provided at home. In-home care consists of formal home care (such as home-delivered meals, e.g., meals on wheels, telephone reassurance, even as long-distance caregiving), adult daycare, respite care, and hospice care (Goldberg, 2014). Institutional care may be provided in continuing care retirement communities, congregate housing, or facilities that include nursing homes and assisted living (Goldberg, 2014).

In India, nursing homes usually refer to some private institutions that provide high-cost medical care. Therefore, long-term care in India is not very distinctly structured as it is in the United States. In India, presently, eldercare services consist of residential care, daycare centers, geriatric care in limited government and non-government institutions, and a few other inspiring activities taken up by some non-governmental organizations sporadically (Ponnuswami & Rajasekaran, 2017). At least at the primary levels, medical care is quite affordable for most people, and in this regard, the country is more generous for its citizens compared to even many other developed countries. Although the types of care are not always accessible because they are scanty in number, the government is trying to build more medical care centers at all primary, secondary, and tertiary levels. However, the scenario is entirely different in long-term care; more education and mass awareness are necessary in order to secure the utilization of available resources more frequently, especially by the older adult population. The uneven disposition of older adults in rural and urban areas and socioeconomic disproportion may be barriers to long-term care utilization. In these circumstances, implementation of a proper long-term care policy involving well-known educators, gerontologists, geriatricians, and nongovernmental organizations should be a government priority.

The US healthcare system is considered one of the best globally. The Centers for Medicare and Medicaid Services (CMS) is constantly working to protect people's health. Since its introduction in 1987, the Omnibus Budget Reconciliation Act

(OBRA) is trying to improve the quality of life of nursing home residents, ensuring maximum services to maintain their best possible physical, mental, and psychosocial well-being (Koren, 2010). In addition, the Affordable Care Act enacted in 2010 targets affordable health insurance to reduce healthcare costs and expand Medicare coverage to a larger population (Rosenbaum, 2011). However, the ultimate goal has not been achieved; the current system of care fails to correspond to the care preferences and needs of many older adult residents (Bartels, 2003).

Although most older adults want to age in place, about 1.4 million residents received care in over 15,000 nursing homes in the United States in the past year (Harris-Kojetin et al., 2016). As nursing homes are one of the main pillars of long-term care in the United States, their services are often scrutinized due to increasing concern about the quality of life and quality of care, from the levels of policymakers, consumers, or researchers (Hansen et al., 2017; Harrington et al., 2001). Although nursing home quality measures have improved a lot in the last few years, the highest level of care is still not received by most residents, possibly due to the care needs of residents in any nursing home continue to become more complex. Quality is a multifaceted term and is influenced by a compound effect of various factors in a nursing home (Hansen et al., 2017). Recently, through the Nursing Home Care website, the CMS facilitates public reporting to inform potential consumers about the quality of care, helping them to compare quality among providers and encourage providers to compete on quality.

Quality of care is vital to improve the quality of life of residents residing in a nursing home (Stadnyk et al., 2011). Although the quality of care in a nursing home depends on several factors, there is a strong association between the overall quality and different proposed quality indicators. Donabedian's structure-process-outcome (SPO) analytical framework is an extensively used model to describe healthcare quality (Donabedian, 1988). The SPO model delineates that in nursing homes, "structural" factors entail physical factors, such as the nursing home's architectural environment and the number and quality of staff. "Process" factors warrant the guidelines for care providers to follow, while delivering the care to residents, whereas "outcome" is evaluated through both objective (e.g., clinical health status) and subjective (e.g., consumers', i.e., residents' and family members' satisfaction) indicators (Spangler et al., 2019). Current research indicates some prominent interconnectedness among these factors, i.e., how "structural" factors (e.g., environmental modifications and the number of staff) and "process" factors (e.g., interpersonal relationships between residents and direct care workers) influence health "outcomes" (Bhattacharyya et al., 2021a; Bowblis & Roberts, 2020).

The current global age-friendly movement targets every individual to become involved in community activities, irrespective of their age, and considers everyone to be worthy of equal respect and dignity. Although the concept of an age-friendly community substantially depends on structural modifications of the community (including home), it also includes changes in interpersonal relationships. According to the World Health Organization (WHO), an age-friendly community involve eight domains of biopsychosocial infrastructure to promote well-being at any age. These domains are housing, social participation, respect and social inclusion, communication and information, community support and health services, civic participation and employment, outdoor spaces and buildings, and transportation (De Biasi et al., 2020). In recent years the WHO took the initiative to include health systems as a part of the age-friendly movement. These eight domains can help guide the development of an age-friendly health system (De Biasi et al., 2020). The current concept of an age-friendly health system consists of four components, which are commonly known as the "4M" model, delineating what *matters* to the concerned individual and institutional care related to *medication, mobility,* and *mentation* (Fulmer et al., 2018). The 4M model places emphasis on the knowledge of fundamentals to provide the best possible care to older adult residents (what *matters* to them), to provide the best level of functionality to maintain their *mobility,* minimizing the side effects of *medications* to help them maintain their quality of life and providing further attention to their cognitive performances, including dementia, delirium, and depression (*mentation*) (Fulmer & Li, 2018).

5.4   Person-Centered Care: Potential and Present Challenges

At later ages, an older adult's healthcare needs often become more complex and chronic. With the changing pattern in lifestyles, residential care needs in long-term care settings, especially the nursing homes, are showing an increasing trend. Due to various psychosocial factors, people are becoming more dependent on formal care. However, an optimal quality of services is not always available; long-term care settings, including nursing homes, could be better at providing maximum services to maintain residents' well-being. Here comes the significance of person-centered care. Person-centered care is a relatively new approach to care that requires the involvement of care partners on the one hand and active participation of the residents themselves on the other. True person-centered care in nursing homes should be more than merely meeting some quality measures (Edelman et al., 2021). According to the Centers for Medicare and Medicaid Services (CMS), person-centered care is "an individualized goal-oriented care plan based on the person's preferences, where care is supported by an inter-professional team in which the person is an integral team member" (CMS, 2017; CMS Ref: Definitions 483.5). Long-term care residents, especially nursing home residents, are usually frail, whose capacity to direct their own daily routine changes due to various chronic conditions. Moreover, every individual is different in their physical character, behavioral and psychological symptoms, and the family and social environments where they lived (Molony et al., 2018). Therefore, the evaluation and the subsequent care approach for every resident should be individualized to maintain their quality of life (Takeda et al., 2012). Although an increasing demand for person-centered care is growing, its fullest implementation and application remains elusive (Bhattacharyya et al., 2021b). Long-term care services and support organizations are experiencing massive staff shortages and instability, especially in the direct care workforce (Bhattacharyya et al., 2021b; Jeon et al., 2012); the post-pandemic situation has created further uncertainty in this sector (Scales, 2021). Recruitment, retention, and training of staff in their healthcare roles are crucial for the proper implementation of person-centered care (Bhattacharyya et al., 2021b). Recognizing and providing high-quality training to nursing home staff are also persistent challenges as nursing home staff have very little time to be exposed to such activities given acuity and workload (Jeon et al., 2012). Direct care workers are a group of workers who struggle the most (Scales, 2021; Scales et al., 2019). They have to take on a variety of responsibilities, which increase their workload and, as a consequence, lead to burnout. In real-life situations, direct care workers need to assist residents in nearly all daily living activities and are often required to do it for an unrealistic number of residents throughout their shift. When asked about the person-centered approach, the direct care workers struggle with understaffing at their workplace, which is neither created by them nor do they have any control to solve the problem (Bhattacharyya et al., 2021b). The most challenging part of their job role is self-motivation. Most supervisors often do not recognize and respect their jobs, their positions, as if they are only working as a stopgap, without what others see as the most fundamental competencies. The frustrations of the direct care workers seem to be the greatest obstacle to successfully implementing person-centered care (Bhattacharyya et al., 2021b). To check this gap in caregiving should be the ultimate responsibility of the institutional authorities. Slight respect and appreciation from the supervisors for the work done by the direct care workers can make the teamwork much better. The direct care workers also have some confusion regarding the extent to which they should allow the residents to satisfy their choices. This dearth of understanding is a big barrier in implementing person-centered care in a nursing home setting and requires education and clear person-centered conversations related to the quality of life, risk, and safety priorities with residents, family, and staff. Limited time and institutional regulations are also barriers to this issue. A caregiver should realize and recognize that it is essential for the individual to do things that give meaning and purpose to the resident's life. For this, they need to understand knowing the person in totality to provide an appropriate environment in the nursing home. For this realization, one needs time; unless a caregiver creates time from the core of their heart, caregiving will remain a mere "facility attendant job," and the goal of person-centered care will not be satisfactory for anyone. On the other hand, higher-level workers, i.e., the supervisors, are mostly administrative personnel. They are often sandwiched. On the one hand, they are deeply concerned about the care of the residents they are supervising, and on the other hand, they are responsible for maintaining the priorities of the nursing home administration, including constraints on staff allowance, personnel costs, and regulatory requirements. Regarding the implementation of person-centered care, they also face the understaffing issue. Compared to the direct care workers, certainly, they are more knowledgeable about the resident's care. Still, somehow their expressions on the values of person-centered care seem similar to the direct care workers (Bhattacharyya et al., 2021b). In a study, Bhattacharyya and colleagues (2021b) found that the nursing home staff of any level needs further training to support the ability of residents to exercise control over their daily lives. Many studies emphasize the basic content of staff training;

however, identifying the interactive methods of training, like a demonstration, role play, intervention delivery in the direct care workers' workplace, and hands-on activities, is still unclear to most staff (Kemeny & Mabry, 2017). Active learning, among either direct care workers or supervising staff members, can be enhanced by ongoing supervision, evaluation, and motivation (Kemeny & Mabry, 2017; Scales et al., 2019). There are some definite facilitators of person-centered care, but currently, the barriers are more in number regarding the successful implementation of person-centered care in long-term care settings (Bhattacharyya et al., 2021b; Scales, 2021).

In most institutional care, the resident management plan generally follows a fixed schedule designed for groups of residents to support healthcare staff to manage care activities; individual treatment plans have not traditionally been the primary focus (Bergman-Evans, 2004). The professionals engaged in resident management in institutional care settings are challenged to apply new thoughts in caregiving due to a mammoth workload within a limited timeframe. However, fresh concepts are required as an alternative management tool that needs awareness generation and ongoing education among the residents and employees (Bergman-Evans, 2004). Another challenge faced by direct care workers is that the older adults often show resistance to learning new skills, and the staff may feel that their current knowledge is under challenge. Often, attempts to modify individual behaviors and organizational care practices become conflicting and usually end in implementing old and traditional practices (Maslow, 2013).

Consumer complaints are often considered a proxy measure of the quality of care and quality of life in long-term care, especially nursing homes. The standardization measures to evaluate and categorize residents' complaints are still not very clear and uniform, though considered necessary. The quality of nursing homes is influenced by different categories of individuals, such as residents, family members, nursing home staff, and administrators (Davis, 1991). The evaluation of every resident is different, and the care approach should be individualized depending on the person's needs and living environment to provide a good quality of care. However, this is not always possible in the practical scenario and rather not maintained in many nursing homes. This gap of caregiving in healthcare settings generates resident dissatisfaction in the long run. According to Bengtson et al. (1997), social constructionist theories of aging focus on the changes of social realities over time, highlighting the necessity to alter individuals' social roles. Therefore, both caregivers and care recipients must reconcile some unavoidable situations that occur in the institutional settings.

To ensure satisfactory care for all institutionalized residents, the Omnibus Budget Reconciliation Act (OBRA) of 1987 has great importance. This act was introduced to enhance the quality of life of nursing home residents to "be provided with services sufficient to attain and maintain his or her highest practicable physical, mental, and psychosocial well-being" (Koren, 2010, p. 312). Although practically, there is a long way to go. Person-centered care should always be directed toward residents; the care staff is also an integral part of this two-way intervention process. The concept of person-centered care is a triangular model (Fig. 5.1), where one end

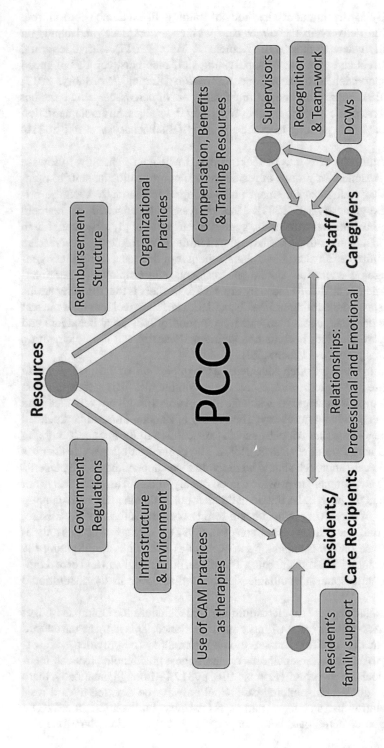

Fig. 5.1 Concept of person-centered care model

focuses on the care-receiver, one end focuses on the caregiver, and the other end directs toward the availability of resources. Person-centered care always focuses on the resident concerned; however, the study by Bhattacharyya and colleagues (2021b) revealed another side of the story, i.e., unless we concentrate equally on the caregiving-staff, their satisfaction and dissatisfaction factors, and the resources available, the person-centered care approach will remain fictitious.

Regarding drawing an association between the age-friendly health system and person-centered care, especially in the nursing home, Fig. 5.1 suggests that the current concept needs some expansion. A person-centered, individualized approach to engagement requires culture change at the organizational level to systematically transform practices of staff, residents, and other care partners. Often, when attempts to change individual behaviors and organizational care practices become very difficult, the nursing home falls back on traditional practices (Best et al., 2012). The current 4M model of age-friendly health system focuses only on the residents; however, it does not specifically address every component of caregiving in a nursing home environment. Aligning the SPO model in the age-friendly nursing home framework would best guide in implementing person-centered care in nursing homes. More research is necessary to create an all-encompassing age-friendly health system model to incorporate other perspectives of nursing home (or any institutional) care, such as caregivers' job satisfaction and making nursing home administration responsible for providing residents with the best possible quality of life.

5.5   Family Caregiving: A Promising Option

Caregivers are considered essential national healthcare resources. With the advancements in medical management, more people live with chronic illnesses and disabilities. With an obvious consequence of increasing life expectancies, many of us find ourselves caring for a loved one at home, as most individuals want to age in place. Whatever the service we provide, it is evident that engaging in care for a family member with morbidity is an act of kindness, love, and loyalty; we dedicate our minds much more while caring for our family members than whatever service we provide at workplaces. Day after day, we gift our loved ones with our care and attention to enhance their quality of life. For most community-living older adults, families often are the primary source of care and support, contributing services that would cost enormous monetary expenses annually if they had to be purchased from outside. However, research has widely documented that assuming a caregiving role can be stressful and burdensome. Depression and other psychological distress indicators are often linked to poorer physical health (Roth et al., 2018). Moreover, along with the physical and psychological strain on the caregivers over time, it is associated with high levels of unpredictability and produces secondary stress in other aspects of life, such as work and family relationships (Schulz & Sherwood, 2008). Therefore, the idea of merging the family caregiving and workplace sectors would bring a huge benefit to society.

The role of burden in caregivers of medically ill or depressed older adults is particularly based upon disease type and phase of the disease (Wilkins et al., 2020). Furthermore, caregivers' distress level was also associated with the gender of both caregiver and care recipient; it was evident that caregiver burden was greater for family caregivers of men, seemingly related to greater aggressive behaviors in male patients (Wilkins et al., 2020). On the other hand, caregivers' reward in predicting lower patient depression scores signals a potential protective factor of caregiver reward on the care recipient; for instance, female patients have been found to be more socialized to express gratitude and appreciation to caregivers than male patients, having an impact on reducing the stress of caregiving (Wilkins et al., 2020). It has been found that family caregiving, like other prosocial helping behaviors, provides stress-buffering adaptations to ameliorate the impact of stress on deteriorating health outcomes, e.g., mortality (Roth et al., 2018).

It could be viewed from a different context. During the past century, a significant gender shift among older adults aged 65+ years took place in the United States, from 108.5 (in 1900) to 79.7 (in 2017) men for every 100 women. These dramatic shifts in numbers, especially over the past few decades, left more women living alone and widowed, contrary to men who more likely remained married or attended by women (Jurkowski, 2018, p.8). The introduction of females into the workforce has led to some important modifications in socioeconomic structures. The families where women entered the workforce have shown a substantial increase in family income (Birkland, 2020, p.42). However, median family income among families where the wife stays at home remained stagnant. Although US policy does not change radically as most people do not support such rapid change, this has brought about profound policy implications (Birkland, 2020, p.99). Besides childcare, women gradually contribute to the care of a partner, parents, parents-in-law, or other family members in need of care because of poor health, age-related issues, or just as a family responsibility. Women as family caregivers are the pivot in maintaining the health and quality of life of individuals who need care (Ehrlich et al., 2020). Ensuring women's income as monetary compensation for family caregiving may enhance the families' socioeconomic status. The basic concept of the proposal to pay family caregivers is multidimensional; still, if we need to pick the most important one, highlighting the economic status improvement at the individual, family, and society level would be the most prominent one. Simultaneously, policymakers must ensure that the proposal of paying family caregivers should not be misused; the primary idea of the proposal, i.e., caring for helpless older adults, does not remain neglected.

Diseases related to lifestyle are showing an increasing trend and are considered a major public health concern. As many individuals desire to age in place, they do not want to readjust themselves, especially in an environment they are not much familiar with. Thus, caregiving often becomes trivialized in the perspectives of personal autonomy and person-centered care goals; interpersonal relations are gradually transforming into mechanical ones. Institutional caregiving in later life brings only two options to most of us: for the diseased individual, either medical care or social care, and for family members, either devote time for caring for a loved one or spend an enormous amount of money. Family caregiving, when compensated with monetary support, brings a balance between the two for everyone.

5.6   COVID-19: Challenges on Caregiving

Many studies suggested that historical transitions and big societal events cumulatively affected individual development, ultimately related to health outcomes. In recent years, socioeconomic inequality has emerged as one of the central focuses of health in aging research. Aging is now considered not just as a segregated process, rather a continuous process that starts from even before birth. The factors associated with health, i.e., physical, psychological, social, environmental, and spiritual well-being, impact people to acquire their individuality cumulatively throughout their life. Globalization through export-import, media publicity, and immigration pattern continuously changes the stabilities in any sector throughout the world. Therefore, the current blow of the pandemic should not be viewed only as a challenge on the healthcare sector of the United States but also as a threat to the social structure of the United States as a complex, dependent, and ongoing process linked with the entire world. No country could isolate itself socioeconomically; this is a bidirectional cumulative inequality affecting individual, societal, and country levels.

The current pandemic has brought a completely different scenario in the sector of caregiving. It is already estimated that older adults, aged 65 years or older, accounted for 81% of US pandemic deaths (Burling, 2021). On the one hand, the COVID-19 pandemic has added more strain on the caregivers; on the other hand, it reduced the quality of care and quality of life (Zimmerman et al., 2020). In family caregiving, the pandemic enhances chances of long-distance caregiving, while in long-term settings, it has compounded the care needs of residents living with multiple health complexities, and demand for direct care is increasing (Scales, 2021; Scales & Lepore, 2020). However, due to uncertainty in recruiting and retaining direct care staff during a pandemic, long-term care facilities, including nursing homes, are experiencing worse staffing shortages than before the pandemic (Quinton, 2020; Scales, 2021). Despite having minimal training, many direct care workers suddenly realize they are essential (Scales, 2021; Scales & Lepore, 2020). Without providing sustained support for this workforce, employers will continue to experience high turnover rates and persistent loss of caregiving staff, especially direct care workers, to other sectors with better benefits (Scales & Lepore, 2020). Inadequate staffing forces direct care workers to prioritize the care tasks for the people they are caring for. This unprecedented scenario in long-term care, especially in nursing home care, underscores the importance of the pre-pandemic findings. Family caregiving could be beneficial for both caregivers and care recipients to minimize economic hardship in many ways. On the other hand, nursing home residents are a high-risk group due to age, chronic disease burden, and congregate living. Both social distancing and personal protective equipment reduce the threat of COVID-19 and increase the possibility for increased social disengagement for an already vulnerable population (Zimmerman et al., 2020). This is also true from the caregivers' perspective, making them vulnerable to social disengagement and susceptible to infection, indirectly increasing economic expenses in many ways. Family caregiving could be advantageous in many ways for both caregivers and care recipients to minimize economic hardship and to maintain more social engagement. However, scrutinizing the impact of caregiving largely depends on intraindividual differences; the association of caregiving and health is a complex issue and largely depends on the concerned individual's outlook.

5.7 COVID-19: Impact on Medicare, Social Security, and Disability

The caregiving sector is also facing a threat by the indirect impact of the pandemic. It is difficult to estimate new areas of potential COVID-related Medicare costs that are not considered yet. It is expected that researchers will go on exploring the impact of the pandemic on the recent past and compare various data with the pre-pandemic situation, leading to a lot of academic publications; however, those would not provide major relief to the national system as the whole system is suffering. This is a problem currently faced by almost the entire world. The fact is that it is our total failure that we have not prepared for such a disaster, and we did not have a "plan B" ready to overcome this devastating situation. Furthermore, we also need to change our focus on various other areas, such as social security, which is probably the most sensitive item in the federal budget that was established in 1935. The program provides a great resource for older adults and the disabled and insurance protection to a large group of people who work in wage and salary jobs and are self-employed (Jurkowski, 2018, p.105). It is already proven for many as a demarcating resource between having a home and homelessness. The global inclination for privatization poses a risk to many countries. This has already been proven historically that any transition to privatization must overcome various major financial hurdles. The Social Security fund has already accumulated an enormous amount of dollars in liabilities to those workers either already retired or will retire soon. However, with the passage of time, people drawing social security will increase as a proportion of the overall working population (Birkland, 2020, p.44). Privatization needs to go through a long and complex process, which, on the one hand, needs funds to pay for these liabilities but, on the other hand, needs enough money from young workers to deposit in new private accounts. This will either require borrowing or a new federal tax load for the general population; otherwise, this will run under huge deficits. A single-headed public system will be guided by different individuals and companies, thus making it more confusing for the general population. This fund will then regulate the whole economic system instead of being regulated by the economic system and thus may engulf many other federal systems. The workers will remain only as apparent decision-makers, but some dishonest businessmen will siphon the profit. Overall, this may reduce national savings. This may ultimately create some distinct social classes, which is nothing but an initial step to creating turmoil in any democracy. Though private retirement accounts may have some significance to attain a change over time, privatization of the present "pay-as-you-go retirement system," whether it is partial or full, would bring only complexities; policymakers should take careful steps on this sensitive issue. Somehow, the pandemic poses a subtle threat to various national systems.

COVID-19 reduced many elective medical visits for the general population due to lockdown and associated fear. However, these enhanced emergency hospitalizations, and subsequent huge expenses forced many healthcare institutions to obtain federal loans from the Medicare fund. Its continuity depends largely on how those loan amounts are recollected (Burling, 2021). Due to the long closure of Social Security offices and reduced staffing as people worked remotely, disability applications became more difficult. People who became more anxious about running out of money also became more pessimistic about saving, leading to a threat of future retirement trouble (Burling, 2021). Furthermore, the whole process may drop in payments for affected beneficiaries. High turnover, stepdown, and unemployment are expected to impose a significant long-term effect on social security and Medicare. Apparently, it seems that early deaths of many older adults will provide some relief to Medicare and Social Security budgets. Although many experts still think that the COVID-related changes would not have much effect on Social Security, this is not yet established. The current pandemic will create turmoil in the national system, not only in the United States but also globally in the long run. Maybe we are currently experiencing the tip of the iceberg; the real disaster is yet to come.

5.8 End-of-Life Care: The Current Scenario

Faith and spirituality have important and powerful roles in the functioning of healthcare today. It is not very rare to find healthcare professionals to address prayer and other religious and spiritual practices, either in visible or invisible ways. This practice is true from the perspective of any country. Though modern medicalization and the "death business" already have emerged as black clouds on humanity, still superiority of emotions exists as the only hope. Most caregivers feel uncomfortable with "torturing" the patients with aggressive treatment to elongate their lives. Death causes tremendous exhaustion for the dying person during their transition phase (transition from life to death). At the same time, the concerned death also causes exhaustion to the surrounding persons, especially after prolonged caregiving in a terminal illness, and more so to those who regularly work in this environment for people of diverse religious traditions. This impact is a professional hazard.

Hospice is a kind of palliative care emerging in the field of end-of-life care. The book chapter "What are Hospice and Palliative Care" is a detailed description of care during the last phase of life by Stephen Connor (2009). Still, there is confusion regarding these types of demarcation in end-of-life care. Hospice provides nearly all support and care required for a person in their end stage of life to ease death. Practically do we not try to give comfort as much as possible for our beloved dying ones, who are not in hospice? On the other hand, if we do not do this for our dearest ones, how can a professional caregiver arrange maximum comfort for a stranger? Especially in a setting where the "requirement of prognosis" is not a criterion.

Currently, hospice service is an emerging business in different parts of the globe. Nursing homes are already proven to be a profitable business setting for a long while. So why not combine these two? Business-minded people are gaining double profit from this coexistence. On the other hand, researchers are analyzing that nursing homes must increase minimum nursing staff only in order to smooth the running of the nursing homes with increased hospice services and get additional staff hours at a minimal cost. Care recipients are gaining apparent comfort, and the issues like death, dying, and loss become only the second issue for discussion. This concept is a pragmatic way to show how everything is engulfed by the materialistic world.

A movement regarding palliative care has just been initiated, and in most parts of the world, the concept of palliative care is either scattered or nonexistent. Even in those countries that remain in the upper portion of the list, much work needs to be done. India and China, the two largest populated countries, are ranked near the bottom of the list regarding the quality of death index. In India, the stage is not prepared for the acceptance of palliative care. The societal structure is very diverse and complex there. Only one state, Kerala, in the southern part of the country, shows some acceptance. Even experts are worried that there is very little chance of it to spread. We are much more focused on the battles against infant, child, and maternal mortality and safe sanitation. Though the population explosion is overwhelming as a black cloud in our progression, we are still surprisingly silent on this matter.

In the United States, Medicare (insurance) bears most of the reimbursements in hospice services. Still, there exists a racial disparity in this domain regarding its usage. Lepore et al. (2011) described in their article "Hospice Use Among Urban Black and White US Nursing Home Decedents in 2006" how hospice use is lower in Black Americans compared to White Americans. The authors pointed to the fear of undertreatment and low quality of care among Black Americans as the most common causes of their lower enrollment in hospice. It seems the lack of awareness in this segment of care and the complexity of medical care regulations in the United States are also responsible for this lower enrollment. The reduction of racial differences in hospice use is not an easy task, and it will take much time for the targeted group of people to be accustomed to it. Though its core values seem to be cross-culturally similar, like midwifery or the idea of an afterlife, cultural beliefs still are too strong for older adults to accept anything. The myth that if one goes in, (s)he will not be able to come out is not only believed by any particular age group; instead, this also is deeply rooted in life thoughts (maybe in genes!) of conservative societies for generation after generation. Most people experience a spiritual feeling after attaining a certain age, and the belief that "end-of-life pain" will probably be a test of trust in God is not only limited to the African Americans but also universal. Almost all ancient civilizations possess that thought (at least as per my limited readings and knowledge). The percentage varies according to the life course and environment. Therefore, we have to generate awareness, not only among African Americans but also worldwide, regarding the concept of hospice (and end-of-life care). Still, the confusion will persist (probably forever) about who is correct and who is not.

5.9 Conclusion

In Hinduism, death is considered a transition to the next life until *moksha* (ultimate destination of the soul to reunite with our source) is achieved. This transition depends on our past works (*karma*). If we do good works, these lead us toward good death (and subsequently good rebirth), and bad works lead us toward bad death (and subsequently bad rebirth). Thus, in ancient times, people practiced "Sanyas" (complete detachment from the mundane world) in their last quarter of life to make this transition as sacred as possible. They refused to take any medications to attain morally immaculate souls and wanted to feel pain as their punishment for past sins. I do not know if there is a contradiction of these thoughts or not and if the enhancement of "comfort and quality of life" in end-of-life care has any influence on pre-death or afterdeath conditions. In India, apparently, terms like *hospice* and *palliative care* are not very common. There are very few organizations providing this type of care compared to many other so-called developed countries. Still, the concept is not uncommon. There is a place called "Moksha Bhawan" (salvation home) in Varanasi. Probably this was the first of its kind in the entire world, established in the early 1920s. Situated on the bank of the holy river "the Ganges," people come here who are expected to die within 15 days (though they often allow them to stay longer).

References

Bartels, S. J. (2003). Improving the system of care for older adults with mental illness in the United States. *The American Journal of Geriatric Psychiatry, 11*(5), 486–497. https://doi.org/10.1176/appi.ajgp.11.5.486

Bengtson, V. L., Burgess, E. O., & Parrott, T. M. (1997). Theory, explanation, and a third generation of theoretical development in social gerontology. *The Journals of Gerontology. Series B, Psychological Sciences and Social Sciences, 52*(2), S72–S88. https://doi.org/10.1093/geronb/52b.2.s72

Bergman-Evans, B. (2004). Beyond the basics. Effects of the Eden Alternative model on quality of life issues. *Journal of Gerontological Nursing, 30*(6), 27–34. https://doi.org/10.3928/0098-9134-20040601-07

Best, A., Greenhalgh, T., Lewis, S., Saul, J. E., Carroll, S., & Bitz, J. (2012). Large-system transformation in health care: A realist review. *The Milbank Quarterly, 90*(3), 421–456. https://doi.org/10.1111/j.1468-0009.2012.00670.x

Bhattacharyya, K. K., Molinari, V., & Hyer, K. (2021a). Self-reported satisfaction of older adult residents in nursing homes: Development of a conceptual framework. *The Gerontologist*, gnab061. Advance online publication. https://doi.org/10.1093/geront/gnab061

Bhattacharyya, K. K., Morgan, J. C., & Burgess, E. O. (2021b). Person-centered care in nursing homes: Potential of complementary and alternative approaches and their challenges. *Journal of Applied Gerontology*, 7334648211023661. Advance online publication. https://doi.org/10.1177/07334648211023661

Birkland, T. A. (2020). *An introduction to the policy process* (5th ed.). Routledge. ISBN: 978-1-351-02394-8.

Bowblis, J. R., & Roberts, A. R. (2020). Cost-effective adjustments to nursing home staffing to improve quality. *Medical Care Research and Review, 77*(3), 274–284. https://doi.org/10.1177/1077558718778081

Burling, S. (2021). *Social Security and Medicare may experience their own COVID-19 side effects, experts say there could be bad news for people who turned 60 last year. Some long haulers may also consider disability.* Retrieved on March 7, 2021, from: https://www.inquirer.com/health/coronavirus/how-will-covid-19-affect-social-security-medicare-disability-20210301.html

Carter, R., & Golant, S. K. (1994). *Helping yourself help others: A book for caregivers.* Times Books. ISBN 978-0812925913.

Connor, S. R. (2009). *Hospice and palliative care: The essential guide* (2nd ed.). Routledge.

Davis, M. A. (1991). On nursing home quality: A review and analysis. *Medical Care Review, 48*(2), 129–166. https://doi.org/10.1177/002570879104800202

De Biasi, A., Wolfe, M., Carmody, J., Fulmer, T., & Auerbach, J. (2020). Creating an age-friendly public health system. *Innovation in Aging, 4*(1), igz044. https://doi.org/10.1093/geroni/igz044.

Donabedian, A. (1988). The quality of care: How can it be assessed? *JAMA, 260*(12), 1743–1748. https://doi.org/10.1001/jama.260.12.1743

Edelman, L. S., Drost, J., Moone, R. P., Owens, K., Towsley, G. L., Tucker-Roghi, G., & Morley, J. E. (2021). Applying the age-friendly health system framework to long term care settings. *The Journal of Nutrition, Health & Aging, 25*(2), 141–145. https://doi.org/10.1007/s12603-020-1558-2

Ehrlich, U., Möhring, K., & Drobnič, S. (2020). What comes after caring? The impact of family care on women's employment. *Journal of Family Issues, 41*(9), 1387–1419. https://doi.org/10.1177/0192513X19880934

Ferraro, K. F., & Shippee, T. P. (2009). Aging and cumulative inequality: How does inequality get under the skin? *The Gerontologist, 49*(3), 333–343. https://doi.org/10.1093/geront/gnp034

Fulmer, T., & Li, N. (2018). Age-friendly health systems for older adults with dementia. *The Journal for Nurse Practitioners, 14*(3), 160–165. https://doi.org/10.1016/j.nurpra.2017.09.001

Fulmer, T., Mate, K. S., & Berman, A. (2018). The age-friendly health system imperative. *Journal of the American Geriatrics Society, 66*(1), 22–24. https://doi.org/10.1111/jgs.15076

Goldberg, T. H. (2014). The long-term and post-acute care continuum. *The West Virginia Medical Journal, 110*(6), 24–30.

Hansen, K. E., Hyer, K., Holup, A. A., Smith, K. M., & Small, B. J. (2017). Analyses of complaints, investigations of allegations, and deficiency citations in United States. *Medical Care Research and Review, 76*(6), 736–757. https://doi.org/10.1177/1077558717744863

Harrington, C., Woolhandler, S., Mullan, J., Carrillo, H., & Himmelstein, D. U. (2001). Does investor-ownership of nursing homes compromise the quality of care? *International Journal of Health Services, 32*(2), 315–325. https://doi.org/10.2190/EBCN-WECV-C0NT-676R

Harris-Kojetin, L., Sengupta, M., Park-Lee, E., Valverde, R., Caffrey, C., Rome, V., & Lendon, J. (2016). Long-term care providers and services users in the United States: Data from the National Study of Long-Term Care Providers, 2013-2014. Vital & Health Statistics. Series 3, *Analytical and Epidemiological Studies,* (38), x–105.

Jeon, Y. H., Luscombe, G., Chenoweth, L., Stein-Parbury, J., Brodaty, H., King, M., & Haas, M. (2012). Staff outcomes from the caring for aged dementia care resident study (CADRES): A cluster randomised trial. *International Journal of Nursing Studies, 49*(5), 508–518. https://doi.org/10.1016/j.ijnurstu.2011.10.020

Jurkowski, E. T. (2018). *Policy and program planning for older adults and people with disabilities* (2nd ed.). Springer Publishing. ISBN 978-0-8261-2839-3.

Kemeny, M. E., & Mabry, J. B. (2017). Making meaningful improvements to direct care worker training through informed policy: Understanding how care setting structure and culture matter. *Gerontology & Geriatrics Education, 38*(3), 295–312. https://doi.org/10.1080/02701960.2015.1103652

Koren, M. J. (2010). Person-centered care for nursing home residents: The culture-change movement. *Health affairs (Project Hope), 29*(2), 312–317. https://doi.org/10.1377/hlthaff.2009.0966

Lepore, M. J., Miller, S. C., & Gozalo, P. (2011). Hospice use among urban Black and White U.S. nursing home decedents in 2006. *The Gerontologist, 51*(2), 251–260. https://doi.org/10.1093/geront/gnq093

Maslow, K. (2013). Person centered care for people with dementia: Opportunities and challenges. *Generations, 37*(3), 8–15.

Molony, S. L., Kolanowski, A., Van Haitsma, K., & Rooney, K. E. (2018). Person-centered assessment and care planning. *The Gerontologist, 58*(Suppl. 1), S32–S47. https://doi.org/10.1093/geront/gnx173

Ponnuswami, I., & Rajasekaran, R. (2017). Long-term care of older persons in India: Learning to deal with challenges. *International Journal on Ageing in Developing Countries, 2*(1), 59–71.

Poo, A. J. (2016). *The age of dignity: Preparing for the elder boom in a changing America*. The New Press. ISBN: 978-1620972018.

Quinton, S. (2020, May 18). *Staffing nursing homes was hard before the pandemic*. Now it's even tougher. Stateline. https://www.pewtrusts.org/en/research-and-analysis/blogs/stateline/2020/05/18/staffing-nursing-homes-was-hard-before-thepandemic-now-its-even-tougher

Rosenbaum, S. (2011). The Patient Protection and Affordable Care Act: Implications for public health policy and practice. *Public Health Reports, 126*(1), 130–135. https://doi.org/10.1177/003335491112600118

Roth, D. L., Brown, S. L., Rhodes, J. D., & Haley, W. E. (2018). Reduced mortality rates among caregivers: Does family caregiving provide a stress-buffering effect? *Psychology and Aging, 33*(4), 619–629. https://doi.org/10.1037/pag0000224

Scales, K. (2021). It's time to resolve the direct care workforce crisis in long-term care. *The Gerontologist, 61*(4), 497–504. https://doi.org/10.1093/geront/gnaa116

Scales, K., & Lepore, M. J. (2020). Always essential: Valuing direct care workers in long-term care. *The Public Policy and Aging Report, 30*(4), 173–177. https://doi.org/10.1093/ppar/praa022

Scales, K., Lepore, M. J., Anderson, R. A., McConnell, E. S., Song, Y., Kang, B., Porter, K., Thach, T., & Corazzini, K. N. (2019). Person-directed care planning in nursing homes: Resident, family, and staff perspectives. *Journal of Applied Gerontology, 38*(2), 183–206. https://doi.org/10.1177/0733464817732519

Schulz, R., & Sherwood, P. R. (2008). Physical and mental health effects of family caregiving. *The American Journal of Nursing, 108*(9 Suppl), 23–27. https://doi.org/10.1097/01.NAJ.0000336406.45248.4c

Spangler, D., Blomqvist, P., Lindberg, Y., & Winblad, U. (2019). Small is beautiful? Explaining resident satisfaction in Swedish nursing home care. *BMC Health Services Research, 19*, 886. https://doi.org/10.1186/s12913-019-4694-9

Stadnyk, R. L., Lauckner, H., & Clarke, B. (2011). Improving quality of care in nursing homes: What works? *Canadian Medical Association Journal, 183*(11), 1238–1239. https://doi.org/10.1503/cmaj.110789

Takeda, M., Tanaka, T., Okochi, M., & Kazui, H. (2012). Nonpharmacological intervention for dementia patients. *Psychiatry and Clinical Neurosciences, 66*(1), 1–7. https://doi.org/10.1111/j.1440-1819.2011.02304.x

The Centers for Medicare and Medicaid Services. (2017). State Operations Manual: Guidance to surveyors for long term care facilities. Retrieved on March 7, 2021, from: https://www.cms.gov/Regulations-and-Guidance/Guidance/Manuals/downloads/som107ap_pp_guidelines_ltcf.pdf

Wilkins, V. M., Sirey, J. A., & Bruce, M. L. (2020). Caregiver reward and burden: Differing constructs in family members providing care for medically ill homebound older adults. *Journal of Aging and Health, 32*(5-6), 361–370. https://doi.org/10.1177/0898264319825760

Zhan, H. J., Liu, G., & Guan, X. (2006). Willingness and availability: Explaining new attitudes toward institutional elder care among Chinese elderly parents and their adult children. *Journal of Aging Studies, 20*, 279–290.

Zimmerman, S., Sloane, P. D., Katz, P. R., Kunze, M., O'Neil, K., & Resnick, B. (2020). The need to include assisted living in responding to the COVID-19 pandemic. *Journal of the American Medical Directors Association, 21*(5), 572–575. https://doi.org/10.1016/j.jamda.2020.03.024

Chapter 6
Aging and Mental Health

6.1 Mental Health Problems: Prevalence

It is still debatable whether prevalence rates of psychiatric disorders show an increasing or decreasing trend in older ages (Reynolds et al., 2015). Some scholars found that mental health problems increase (Beekman et al., 1995) at later ages, whereas according to some studies, they decrease (Reynolds et al., 2015). Regardless of this trend, with constant upward propensity patterns in demographics, geropsychologists and other mental health professionals are expected to manage a higher number of older adults (Petkus & Wetherell, 2013).

Chronic health conditions may cause impaired physical functioning and increased dependence among adults in later life. This condition may be further responsible for the gradual rise in stress levels among older adults. Psychological issues, such as adjustment problems, helplessness due to cognitive decline, spousal caregiving, bereavement, and social role transitions, such as retirement and loss of mastery or family leadership, further aggravate the stress. These all have a conglomerate negative impact on the individuals' health and functional status that directly affects their quality of life. These age-related biopsychosocial complexities have a strong negative feedback effect on psychiatric morbidity, making the diagnosis of mental health problems and their management more cumbersome.

Although the overall prevalence rates of mental health problems such as affective disorders, anxiety disorders, serious mental illness (SMI), and personality disorders increase, older adults receive low rates of psychiatric treatment (Petkus & Wetherell, 2013; Wang et al., 2005). Even when these individuals receive treatment, they are most likely to receive pharmacological management instead of evidence-based psychotherapies (Gum et al., 2010). Moreover, when receiving treatment, most of them are not treated in the community but are hospitalized instead. From the perspective of older adults in need of mental health treatment, there may be a dearth of knowledge about when and where to get the desired management (Petkus & Wetherell,

© The Author(s), under exclusive license to Springer Nature Switzerland AG 2021   59
K. K. Bhattacharyya, *Rethinking the Aging Transition*,
https://doi.org/10.1007/978-3-030-88870-1_6

2013) and the stigma associated with it (Livingston & Boyd, 2010). They possess a reluctant attitude toward psychotherapy from a negative feeling and believe it is a violation of their privacy. The dearth of resources, such as transportation and financial hardship, may also contribute to negative social factors for utilizing therapeutic resources. On the other hand, from the caregivers' perspective, a systemic lack of training among geropsychologists may be a contributing factor (Petkus & Wetherell, 2013). Furthermore, many organic changes resulting from various mental health problems are often seen as part of normal aging and underestimate the prevalence of mental health problems of older adults in the community (Petkus & Wetherell, 2013). Clinicians sometimes want to avoid complex aging issues; sometimes ageism and therapeutic nihilism also play a role in this regard.

Traditional management of mental health issues, irrespective of various government and nongovernmental facilities, may apply a "one-size-fits-all" approach to improve care, while dismissing the idea that individuals differ in treatment needs. Unfortunately, most of these persons often represent complete anosognosia, i.e., they are unaware of their own mental health status. Many clinicians cannot rectify that; by focusing on the deficits, they may unintentionally and wrongfully communicate that the person has declined and is of no value in society. The current person-centered approach shifts the focus from the traditional medical model to a promising social model of care. This approach focuses on the individual's remaining positive sides instead of focusing on the deficits (Power, 2010). The idea of a person-centered approach is utilized to capture one's life story better, enhancing the quality of life, activity engagement level, values, preferences, and lowering stigma associated with the disease. By recognizing this approach, clinicians can develop positive relationships with persons with mental health disorders, especially dementia, better assess and treat these individuals, and assist other formal and informal caregivers.

A vast body of research established that psychotherapy effectively helps individuals cope with various mental health disabilities and helps them function at a nearly optimal level of well-being. As non-pharmacological psychotherapeutic interventions, the four techniques of psychotherapies that are commonly used are behavioral therapy, psychoanalysis, cognitive-behavioral therapy (CBT), and family/systems therapy. Even though the approaches are unique in their nature regarding outcomes, they have many overlapping features. The current discussion will highlight the nature of the four broad geropsychiatric diagnostic categories, such as affective disorders, anxiety disorders, SMI, and personality disorders among older adults that will help understand some critical distinctions between onset and types of various mental health problems. This review will also discuss the four primary management strategies, i.e., behavioral therapy, psychoanalysis, CBT, and systems therapy, for treating those disorders with a specific emphasis on their strengths and limitations with implications and future directions for research in this domain.

6.2   Common Mental Health Issues in Older Adults

6.2.1   Affective Disorders

6.2.1.1   Depression

Depression is, perhaps, the most common mental health problem among older adults; it seems, currently, the medicalization of behavioral health issues remains incomplete without incorporating depression (Kanter et al., 2008). The term came from the Latin word *depressare* or *deprimere*, where *de* means "down" and *premere* denotes "to press," therefore, having a literal meaning of press down. A wide range of symptoms may come under the heading of depression, and this, in fact, creates confusion among both clinicians and the general population. Being metaphorical, "depression" is not used as a technical term (Kanter et al., 2008). Sadness and loss of interest or "anhedonia" are the most familiar symptoms, whereas weight and appetite change, sleep change, agitation, loss of energy, and recurrent thoughts about death also prevail. Older adults with depression often complain about sudden onset memory problems and have earlier depressive episodes. Research suggests that depression rates among community-dwelling older adults are similar to that of younger adults dwelling in the community. Interestingly, the prevalence of depression is higher among institutionalized older adults than those living in the community (Mitchell et al., 2011). Depression is considered a significant comorbidity of various chronic medical conditions. Research suggests that along with the illness itself and the rising medical cost, unsatisfactory quality of care and poor relationship with caregivers are the contributing factors for depression (Wang et al., 2017). However, the actual prevalence of depression is still debatable among the community and compares the institutionalized older adults with those living in the community. As a disorder, depression may show a unipolar and a bipolar variety. While a common depressive symptom is a sadness, many older adults claim not to have any sad feelings, which creates further confusion among clinicians. An older adult with a unipolar variety often complains of loss of memory and lack of concentration.

6.2.1.2   Bipolar Disorder

Bipolar disorder is a chronic mental health issue characterized by extreme shifts in mood, energy, and activity levels, ranging from depressive episodes to manic highs. Manic episodes usually present with euphoria or irritability, sleeplessness, and uncontrollable impulses (Driessen & Hollon, 2010). The disease shows a higher prevalence of cognitive decline and decreased quality of life (Bonnín et al., 2019). Bipolar disorder is usually diagnosed at an early age, though subclinical cases remain undiagnosed until later life. It has been found that individuals with treated bipolar disorder often can maintain high-level leadership positions (Molinari, 2020a).

6.2.1.3 Sleep Disturbance/Insomnia

The idea for the three-part day was introduced on May 1, 1886, in Chicago, Illinois, to offer some welcome respite for industrial workers claiming 8 h of work, 8 hours of recreation, and 8 h of rest. It was one of the earliest movements starting the international tradition of May Day, responsible for probably the biggest ever international policy change. Looking at these three elements, it seems that the scientific community would still support that we need to rest for up to 8 h per day. Evidence widely suggests that our daily performance and long-term general health seem to benefit from 6 to 8 h of sleep every night. Insomnia is a common sleep problem presented by inadequate quality and quantity of sleep, which usually affects adults and older adults (Mai & Buysse, 2008). Insomnia in later life may endanger individuals' daily living with negative health consequences, such as cardiovascular problems (Troxel et al., 2010), progression to dementia (Sindi et al., 2018), low quality of life, the risk for falls, and mortality (Mai & Buysse, 2008). Sleep disorders are among the main adverse effects of depression and late-life anxiety, though many other factors play a role here. This is a significant issue in contemporary society, as most people believe that a substantial reduction in sleep is associated with aging. They fail to recognize the real scenario because of this stigmatization, which repudiates the fact that sleep quality can be improved through cognitive functioning.

6.2.1.4 Involutional Melancholia

Involutional melancholia is comparatively an uncommon mental health problem manifested by slow progression, with onset occurring earlier for women (40–55 years) than men (50–65 years). It has been found that sex hormones play a significant role in developing this disorder. The symptoms range from severe anxiety, agitation, restlessness, and nihilistic delusions to insomnia, anorexia, weight loss, and, ultimately, depression. There is a feeling of guilt, but without having manic features. Due to the absence of the specific diagnostic criteria of this disorder, associated with much overlapping of symptoms, the true cases often remain undiagnosed. Therefore, the actual picture of the prevalence of involutional melancholia in society, compared to major depression, always remains a guesstimate. Even regarding its treatment, if we focus on hormone replacement therapy instead of commonly used antidepressants or mood elevators, the results are not fully answered.

6.2.2 Anxiety Disorders

6.2.2.1 Generalized Anxiety Disorders

Anxiety disorders are also prevalent in later ages, though usually they show a chronic pattern. Anxiety disorders may significantly reduce individuals' productivity and increase caregivers' attention, which ultimately leads to significant societal and economic burdens. Thirty to 40% of anxiety disorders are hereditary (Miloyan et al., 2014). Anxiety disorders become less prevalent after middle age and in older adulthood. Older adults report fewer anxiety symptoms; furthermore, these symptoms are less severe than those reported by their younger counterparts. However, in terms of clinical significance, older adults appear to be more vulnerable to disability. Therefore, even though older adults report a fewer number of and less severe symptoms of anxiety, the symptoms might be responsible for producing clinically significant levels of disability (Miloyan et al., 2014). High levels of distress further aggravate the level of anxiety. Late-life anxiety was found to be frequently associated with depression, cognitive decline, dementia, general medical conditions, and caregiving responsibilities; this reduces life satisfaction, impairs social functioning, and lowers quality of life (Miloyan et al., 2014). Generalized anxiety disorder is the most common anxiety disorder found in later life. Generalized anxiety disorder's typical symptoms expressed by older adults are fear, worry, avoidance, restlessness, fatigue, concentration problems, irritability, and sleep disturbance (Gale & Davidson, 2007; Gum et al., 2010). Although there are some diagnostic ambiguities in identifying specific anxiety disorders due to the coexisting symptom dimensions, the most common symptoms presented by older adults are worries and health conditions, especially in interpersonal relationships and functional disabilities. Various anxiety disorders in later life may lead to cardiac problems, somatic symptoms, reduced quality of life, higher risk for dementia, and burdensome healthcare costs (Ayers et al., 2015). One question often raised is that among late-life anxiety and executive function, which one is responsible for impacting the other? Do persons with anxiety show poor performance on executive function measures due to excessive fret, sleep disturbance, and restlessness? Or does the growing executive dysfunction prevent one from managing stressful life situations? Without creating a subject for debate, it may be concluded that they both affect one another. Probably the loss of extended multigenerational family structure and unplanned gaining of a few extra years in later life through higher life expectancy factors are the most crucial determinants for late-life anxiety.

6.2.2.2   Obsessive-Compulsive Disorder

Obsessive-compulsive disorder (OCD) is a chronic, catastrophic mental health problem in which individuals have some repetitive and annoying thoughts (obsessions) and feel the urge to perform monotonous routine activities (compulsions), which largely impair general functioning and cause distress (Lack, 2012). The obsessive phase is usually associated with an enormous amount of anxiety, and the subsequent compulsions reduce the associated distress. Common obsessions present with fear of germs or contamination, worries about harm to self or others, and having things be in symmetry and in order. On the other hand, common compulsions include excessive cleaning or hand washing, repeated checking, compulsive counting, confessing, praying, rubbing, and avoidance (Lack, 2012). Although OCD commonly develops in childhood, adolescence, and adulthood, it is seen among older adults in substantial numbers. Almost three-fourths of the individuals with OCD present with other comorbid disorders (Lack, 2012). Research suggested that a significant number of OCD cases remain undiagnosed in the community (Ruscio et al., 2010).

6.2.2.3 Post-Traumatic Stress Disorder

Post-traumatic stress disorder (PTSD) is a psychological issue usually triggered by a potentially traumatic event, either a single event or prolonged exposure in a lifetime. PTSD is usually associated with poor physical health and psychiatric comorbidity (Bisson et al., 2015). There are also a large number of subclinical cases of PTSD in the community. Among older adults aged older than 65 years, 70–90% have been exposed to at least one traumatic event in their lifetime. However, nearly 1.5–4% of older adults are diagnosed with clinical PTSD, and around 7–15% have subclinical PTSD (Kaiser et al., 2019).

6.2.2.4 Phobias and Panic Disorders

Phobias are also widespread mental health issues found in all ages; however, there is great variation in their presentation in different ages. While panic disorders accompany phobia in younger ages, they are commonly associated with safety concerns, primary health events, or severe mental trauma in older ages. Symptoms include avoidance of a situation (phobia) and palpitation and sweating (panic disorders). Phobia may also be associated with other mental disorders, such as mood and other anxiety disorders (Rudaz et al., 2017).

6.2.3 Serious Mental Illness

6.2.3.1 Schizophrenia

Schizophrenia is a complex and chronic psychological condition that presents with a combination of some positive and negative symptoms, including delusions, hallucinations, disorganized behavior, and cognitive disabilities (Patel et al., 2014). It is the most severe form of psychopathology. The underlying feature of this disorder is the inability to realize and express reality. Gradual changes in thinking, mood, and behavioral pattern may cause substantial distress to the affected person. Problems in concentration, memory impairment, and social withdrawal are often associated with it. Due to its complex and overlapping manifestations, schizophrenia is often confused with other mental health disorders. However, late-life schizophrenia often shows fewer functional impairments. Most older adults with schizophrenia (nearly 85%) live in the community and are usually admitted to long-term care facilities due to other medical reasons apparently unrelated to schizophrenia (Molinari, 2020a).

6.2.4   Personality Disorders

Personality disorders are a group of mental problems in which an individual's thinking, feeling, and behavior deviate from the expected average pattern (Ekselius, 2018). Perceptions of the world and expectations about what will happen are often skewed. These disorders are characterized by chronic instabilities across multiple functional domains, such as emotion, cognition, and behavior. Personality disorders invariably start in early life; however, they often remain undiagnosed until later life. Diagnosing personality disorders among older adults can be problematic due to limitations of youth-focused diagnostic criteria, various comorbid mental and physical health problems, and complicated histories. Personality disorders often present a history of stressful life experiences associated with a low quality of life and poor physical health (Ekselius, 2018). Baltes and Baltes' selection, optimization, and compensation (SOC) model best describes assessing the internal strengths of an individual with personality disorder most comprehensively regarding biopsychosocial context rather than focusing only on personality deficits (Molinari et al., 2006). In a person-centered care approach, caregivers and the concerned individual may agree on the selected treatment planning and optimize with adaptivity, which compensates for the individual's negative aspects to help them live in the facility environment.

6.2.5   Neurocognitive Disorders

Neurocognitive disorders are a group of neurological disorders that develop due to cognitive deficits, dementia being the typical example. These may be associated with learning and memory. The person fails to recognize known objects (agnosia) and has poor performance in executive function such as thinking and planning and a deficit in attention and social cognition. Although the affected persons are not developmentally disabled, the impairment causes loss of independence, poor judgment, and motor, behavioral, and psychiatric symptoms. Similar to individuals with personality disorders, individuals with neurocognitive disorders are not flexible enough and unable to interpret their experiences to be accustomed to their late-life situations, especially in long-term care facilities.

6.3   Current Therapeutic Approaches

While managing older adults with psychotherapy, the therapist should build a shared world with the client. Emphasis must be given to the patient's strengths and present concerns, not on their negative past life events. Although various psychotherapies can be done in home and daycare settings, older adults with many severe mental health conditions, such as dementia, schizophrenia, personality disorders, and bipolar disorder, are often required to be admitted to nursing homes (Miller & Rosenheck, 2006).

6.3.1   Behaviorism

Behaviorism is a theoretical approach that emphasizes observable behaviors. The term *behaviorism*, associated with classical conditioning, was probably first associated with Pavlov's dog experiment. This theory posits that all behaviors are learned through the interaction of an individual with environmental stimuli. Behaviors are the actions and manners through which a person reacts with the environment to meet their physical, social, and emotional needs. Behavior consists of three components: when a person receives an environmental stimulus, i.e., antecedent, they react through a behavior that results in a response, i.e., consequence. All behavior is thought to follow an antecedent-behavior-consequence path and two basic learning processes, classical and operant conditioning. Classical conditioning involves learning through prior stimulus history, whereas in operant learning, the behavior is controlled by past behavior consequences. Behavioral approaches do not focus on motives, emotions, or any biological influences for the behavior; they do not evaluate the internal states of mind. Instead, behaviorists start to evaluate people from a relatively blank slate and develop an environmental interaction through conditioning (Segal et al., 2011). Before conducting a behavioral adjustment program, a therapist analyzes the environment in which the behavior takes place. After evaluating the consequences of behavior, they try to identify the paths through which the environment triggers the intended behavior.

Understanding the totality of a behavior is the actual strength of behaviorism; the therapy focuses on some particular behavioral problems within certain contexts and narrows the behavior's scope to understand the environmental stimuli causing that behavior. Also, by promoting behavioral activation, the therapy helps individuals find activities pleasant to them. This activation benefits the individual (Segal et al., 2011). However, according to many scholars, behaviorism is a simplistic approach; the concerning stimulus is only useful in certain favorable conditions.

6.3.1.1   Behavioral Therapy for Depression

Older adults often face the challenge resulting from a lack of environmental encouragement that leads to adjustment problems among individuals (Lewinsohn, 1975). This effect, in turn, further leads to reduced satisfaction and depression. In addition, age-related physical and cognitive decline severely impacts the behavior of older adults. This effect is further aggravated in the individuals living in hospitals or nursing homes that mostly limit their environmental interactions. However, when applied in older adults, behaviorism can impact a wide range of areas, such as social interaction and participation, memory and language, health maintenance, sexual problems, sleep difficulties, and disruptive behaviors (Segal et al., 2011). In this context, behavioral therapy has been proven to effectively manage depression in older adults, even those living in various institutional settings.

Behavioral approaches are often used to treat sleep disturbances. The environment causing sleep disturbance should be assessed first, and subsequently the response of the concerned person to the disturbance should be identified and needs to be changed. Engagement in mindful activities, avoiding daytime naps, and following a daily routine are the ways to address sleep disturbances. In a study on a nationally representative dataset (MIDUS), it has been found that participants experiencing a chronic sleep problem at baseline were more likely to engage in mind-body practice (e.g., yoga) persistently in subsequent waves (Bhattacharyya et al., 2020). The addition of regular yoga exercises in the daily routine of older adults may help achieve improved sleep quality as well as improve the quality of life (Bankar et al., 2013). Therefore, in the context of the stressful contemporary world, health practitioners and policymakers should recognize and promote mind-body intervention (e.g., yoga) as an alternative therapeutic practice that is a potentially viable complement to medical management to maintain the quality of life of an individual. Including yoga in our daily activities may not only improve sleep but also may reduce our stress and perhaps even aggression.

6.3.1.2   Behavioral Therapy for Anxiety Disorders

Behavioral approaches are also used to treat anxiety disorders. Research suggests this strategy helps minimize incontinence among older adult residents with anxiety disorders; therefore, it helps to reduce healthcare costs in many ways (Burgio & Burgio, 1986). When applied to an individual with OCD, behavioral therapy is crucial to identify the specific stimulus or the consequence that needs to be targeted. The idea is to reinforce a specific activity to replace negative thoughts that eventually help eliminate the compulsive activities associated with the disease. Therefore, the person would engage in more meaningful, healthy behaviors without the disruptive thoughts (Segal et al., 2011). Behavioral therapy can also help manage symptoms associated with PTSD that involves a thorough assessment of the concerned person's environment to rectify the stimuli associated with the trauma, thereby altering the response related to the problematic behavior by engaging the individual in meaningful activities (Segal et al., 2011).

6.3.1.3   Behavioral Therapy for Schizophrenia

As persons with schizophrenia do not understand real-world situations, the goal of treatment is to support the individual to realize the real world, helping them reacquire the skills and behaviors. A token economy is a behavioral therapeutic approach found to be effective like exercise in individuals with schizophrenia. Through the token economy, the negative symptoms of schizophrenia, such as social withdrawal, can be altered by increased desirable behaviors, such as social interaction (Gholipour et al., 2012). Accumulating evidence suggests that those with schizophrenia in the community show a better prognosis than those living in the institutional environment (Compton et al., 2016). It has been found that older adults with late-onset schizophrenia show a better prognosis than those with early-onset schizophrenia (Molinari, 2020a).

6.3.2   Cognitive-Behavioral Therapy

Cognitive-behavioral therapy (CBT) is a group of psychosocial approaches to improving mental health (Hofmann et al., 2012). CBT is the approach to modifying behaviors that restructure emotional patterns and cognitive functions such as appraisals. CBT, a relatively new form of psychotherapy, has emerged with some overlapping characteristics with behavioral therapy, though it has some distinct techniques in treatment methods (Kaczkurkin & Foa, 2015). CBT uses laws of learning to restructure behavior; however, this not only focuses on external behaviors but also on the thought processes. Thoughts are considered internal behaviors, and CBT aims to change maladaptive behaviors via changing thoughts. CBT does not evaluate the origin of the symptoms; instead, it emphasizes a multidimensional approach to modify current beliefs and controls over an individual's mood. This strategy helps the therapist identify the cognitive and environmental factors responsible for the concerning behavior, thereby improving functioning and remission of the disease (Hofmann et al., 2012). CBT does not include a historical life perspective; however, understanding someone's life story seems vital, particularly while dealing with older adults. Because every individual is different physically and mentally, every person's psychological and social perspectives differ from those of another; therefore, the care approach should also be individualized. Even in the same individual, it differs with advancing age because in most cases, it is unknown from which point in time the problems appeared and what the root cause is. Therefore, the intervention should be approached accordingly.

The goal of CBT is to modify thinking patterns to restructure maladaptive behaviors, such as negative thinking, black-and-white thinking, and all-or-none thinking (Segal et al., 2011). CBT is the most widely used evidence-based strategy for various mental issues. This therapeutic approach's main strength is its focus on the current thoughts and behaviors and the factors responsible for those thoughts and behaviors. The strength of CBT focuses on the overall strategy of symptom reduction, to change current maladaptive behaviors and those of the future. Furthermore, CBT is time-limited and used for a shorter period than other psychotherapies, ultimately resulting in fewer costs associated with the treatment. The coping skills learned during the therapy help individuals tackle distressing symptoms in their daily activities. However, CBT also has certain limitations. First, CBT only focuses on current problems, not the past issues that may be associated with the current manifestations. Therefore, sometimes the underlying causes may remain undiagnosed. Often, individuals with complex mental issues and broad interpersonal dimensions cannot be explained through CBT. As CBT is most useful for restricted symptoms, it does not address broader problems (Segal et al., 2011). Moreover, some scholars suggest that older adults do not benefit from CBT as much as their younger counterparts because CBT protocols demand higher cognitive functions from older adults, causing more anxiety. Older adults need a more individualized, less complicated approach than traditional CBT.

In CBT, a therapeutic relationship should be supportive and empathetic. However, the care partner should also work from an equal level with their clients. The process is not as easy as it looks. In the contemporary era of globalization, personal ego and "Googling" are enough to destroy the respect and trust in the clinician-patient relationship from either end. Therefore, how can a clinician treat a client while being at the same level? It seems an impossible task from the context of dealing with Indian older adults of both "low education and socioeconomic status" and "high education and socioeconomic status," but from a different perspective. It appears that an "equal expert" is a contradiction in terms. Some experts consider that although the geriatric mental health practitioner has expertise in older adults and mental health, the counselor does not try to take over the client's life. Indeed, the counselor exhibits cultural humility and checks with the client about interpretations about what is going on in the client's life and does not assume an omniscient attitude.

The education and socioeconomic status of the care recipient are very important. For instance, in problem-solving therapy, which is one type of CBT in a therapist's armamentarium, the therapist should fit the treatment to the patient's/client's needs, including effective short-term treatment with more modest goals such as symptomatic improvement versus personality change. The therapist first introduces themselves, establishes their credibility, and shares experiences in treating clients with similar mental health issues. The therapist then starts asking for related information about the client, such as the client's financial stability, health, relationships, and previous history of mental health issues. The therapist then presents a briefing about the nature of the sessions and explains the therapeutic goals, such as overcoming stresses, breaking problems into smaller ones, weighing the pros and cons of various solutions, picking the best strategy that suits the situation, and creating a plan of action. If the client is apparently healthy, educated, belongs to high socioeconomic conditions, and mildly depressed, therefore, from a therapist's perspective, (s)he is "easy to manage." However, it is questionable whether this therapy would have equal effectiveness for a client who is not so "easy to manage."

6.3.2.1   CBT for Depression

CBT is often used to treat varieties of affective disorders. Depression in older adults differs from depression among younger individuals in several ways. CBT is based on the concept that inaccurate negative beliefs and maladaptive information processing are the causes of depression. Therefore, after the correction of maladaptive thinking, acute problems and chances of relapse of the subsequent symptoms will be minimized (Driessen & Hollon, 2010). This learning and normalization concept helps depressed individuals learn various adaptive and complementary skills that help them cope with the conditions with an optimistic mood. This reshaped thinking pattern helps them modify their behaviors for more social engagement and remain active (Driessen & Hollon, 2010).

Bipolar disorder usually presents both mania and depression. CBT is widely used as a therapeutic strategy for both aspects of this disorder. CBT focuses on modifying cognitive functionality in both phases of the disease. By identifying the problematic behavior and teaching the person to control their mood, this technique allows them to intervene and prevent future behaviors associated with these behavioral issues. Since withdrawal symptoms may result in both mania and depression, identifying new ways for the individual to remain engaged constantly in their life, even in these phases, should be given the maximum importance.

6.3.2.2   CBT for Anxiety and Other Phobias

Research has widely demonstrated that CBT is efficacious in treating a variety of anxiety disorders (Hans & Hiller, 2013; Kaczkurkin & Foa, 2015). Exposing the older adult to the stressor stimuli and training with an increased number of adaptive cognitive responses are crucial CBT strategies. According to Craske and Barlow's generalized anxiety disorder treatment manual, over time, individuals learn to change thinking patterns that lead to anxiety (Kaczkurkin & Foa, 2015). Other strategies used to manage anxiety disorders are relaxation training, i.e., relaxation during exposure to a scary stimulus, and cognitive modification training, i.e., learning the identification skills and replacing maladaptive thoughts. CBT is also shown to have more impact on younger individuals than older adults. On the other hand, exposure therapy is considered most beneficial for specific phobias, and exposure can also be used along with cognitive modifying strategies (Kaczkurkin & Foa, 2015). However, a meta-analytic study has shown that a combination of exposure approach with cognitive therapy in individuals with specific phobias did not show a favorable result compared to exposure alone (Wolitzky-Taylor et al., 2008).

6.3.2.3   CBT for Serious Mental Illness (SMI)

CBT approaches are also widely used to address SMI, such as managing the positive and negative symptoms of schizophrenia. The treatment method for persons with schizophrenia emphasizes improving independent functional activities, managing symptoms by reducing daily life stress, and addressing the stigma associated with the disease. The overall goal is to improve and maintain the quality of life and functional well-being of the concerned person by identifying and self-monitoring the proper cognitive and behavioral strategies to manage the associated symptoms (Desai et al., 2010).

6.3.2.4   CBT for Personality Disorders

CBT techniques in managing personality disorders have a huge potential to help the older population. CBT is based on the concept that personality disorders are a combination of maladaptive beliefs about oneself and others, environmental factors associated with effective behavior, and deficiencies in skills to modify proper responding. CBT aims to modify these underlying factors by altering cognitive and behavioral functions, exposure, and skill training (Matusiewicz et al., 2010). A randomized controlled trial with individuals with schizophrenia revealed that the individuals who received regular treatment with cognitive-behavioral skill training performed significantly better social functional activities than individuals who received only regular treatment. The combined treatment group also demonstrated higher cognitive insight and mastery in the learned skills than the control group (Granholm et al., 2005).

6.3.3   Psychoanalytic Therapy

Psychoanalytic therapy is an approach to treat mental disorders based on some theories postulated initially by Sigmund Freud and some therapeutic strategies associated with the unconscious mind. Personality, i.e., how we recognize, experience, and interact with the outer world, is shaped by the conflict between three underlying structures of the mind, i.e., id, superego, and ego (Boag, 2014). While the *id* indicates our unconscious state of mind containing desires and needs, the *superego* denotes the traditional moral values. In contrast, the *ego* works as a mediator between these two and makes rational decisions (Boag, 2014; McLeod, 2019). Psychoanalysis is based on the underlying concept that one's feelings and behaviors are rooted in early life experiences, which were incorporated into an individual's unconscious mind and are relatively beyond one's control. Therefore, psychoanalytic therapy aims to uncover notions and thoughts long buried in the subconscious mind. Psychoanalysts emphasize an individual's early life history and try to modify present and future relational perceptions, such as desires, emotions, behavior, and values.

Psychoanalytic therapy emphasizes how past events affect the present and focus on why a specific behavior occurs and the underlying unconscious factor contributing to it. The main strength of psychoanalytic therapy is its comprehensive nature as it considers both mental and behavioral functions of the individuals from a developmental perspective. Many therapists find this strategy helpful with more challenging and complex personalities because this approach helps the therapist find the broadest perspective on human behavior. Furthermore, psychoanalytic theory focuses on the critical roles of the early years' relationships, helping to identify stressors in the individual's life. Although psychoanalysis has some positive aspects, this therapeutic strategy is not appropriate for all types of mental diseases, like psychotic disorders. Moreover, psychoanalysis is an extensive treatment that requires individuals to invest a considerable amount of time and money for treatment purposes. This extensive treatment requires modifying one's personality that undergirds symptoms to counteract symptom substitution (Molinari, 2020b). It takes a very long time to understand the "whys" of a person's behavior. Psychoanalysis also has loftier goals to change one's personality and one's way of being. Not many can afford such a luxury. Furthermore, this approach neither directly addresses symptoms nor does it provide a prompt solution. However, the greatest flaw of psychoanalytic therapy is that it considers personality development stops at 5 years of age. Research has now demonstrated that personality development continues up to 30 years of age, even at any point in life (Segal et al., 2011). Furthermore, anyone in this contemporary era can use psychoanalysis with a bad intention.

Psychoanalysis theory focuses on joining the nuclear family conflicts to effect change within the individual's personality. However, suppose a psychotherapist uses this approach; how could (s)he know the "why" of behavior without spending much time on the care recipients, especially when (s)he is not taking symptoms as the primary interest into account? In this contemporary era, when a "patient" is considered a "client" to the doctor, this seems very difficult, similar to the overarching concept of person-centered care. People often wonder about the generalizability of psychoanalysis. How the process extracts ideas from an introverted person? Or is it the therapist analyzing the situation and providing multiple interpretations from their own? The significance and trustworthiness of psychoanalysis in the present scenario are also questionable issues. As the process is lengthy, how far could an analyst devote their time for "a" client, particularly when we are aging in a world full of stress and complexities? Furthermore, psychoanalysis has been criticized not only because it is a lengthy, costly process, open only to those in the upper socioeconomic classes, but also because it is based on a Western European Judeo-Christian cultural heritage. Regarding the former point, one can be guided by psychoanalytic thinking but not necessarily employ the insight-oriented couch method of psychoanalytic treatment based on Oedipal dynamics that may arise from a European capitalist model that may be alien to Asian, African, and Muslim societies (V. Molinari, personal communication, September 26, 2020).

6.3.3.1   Psychoanalytic Therapy for Depression

Psychoanalytic therapy is based on understanding the subconscious mental state that controls one's feelings and behaviors. Many therapists consider psychoanalysis to provide depressed individuals with a reduction in symptoms, greater self-awareness, and a higher chance of identifying and correcting the problem (Bleichmar 1996). Psychotherapy, in the form of talk therapy, explores thought patterns and feelings. Once the therapist uncovers an individual's subconscious mental state through discussion, they would better control thoughts and behaviors. On the other hand, Scogin et al. (2005) suggested that brief psychodynamic psychotherapy may be useful as an evidence-based treatment for depression among older adults. This psychotherapy specifically combats depression or the loss of purpose or identity.

6.3.3.2 Psychoanalytic Therapy for Anxiety and Other Phobias

Psychoanalysis is often found to impact those with generalized anxiety disorder as it helps patients be conscious of their within-person conflicts. Psychoanalysts believe that generalized anxiety disorder results from a conflict between an individual's self and ego and possibly from a history of having strict and merciless parents in childhood. The therapy aims to identify the underlying conflicts responsible for the disorder and work on this issue to alter the anxiety-related behaviors to improve social functioning and remove the anxious thought processes (Segal et al., 2011). Experts also found that complete removal of phobia is only possible by identifying and solving the original conflict rooted in the subconscious mind (Garcia, 2017).

6.3.3.3 Psychoanalytic Therapy for SMI

The effects of psychoanalytic strategies in the management of schizophrenia and other SMIs have been disputed. Some studies found positive results (Robbins, 2012), while some did not (Malmberg & Fenton, 2001). On the other hand, schizoid personality disorder (SPD) presents with bizarre behaviors, odd perceptions, and acute social discomfort. Psychoanalytic therapy has been beneficial in treating SPD by building rapport via transference and focusing on the individual's childhood years (Ridenour, 2016). SPD is usually associated with insufficient emotions and affection in early life. Psychoanalysts aim to identify the early experiences and reflections upon the individual to modify the schizoid personality (Ridenour, 2016).

6.3.3.4 Psychoanalytic Therapy for Personality Disorders

Research has also found that psychoanalysis is an effective strategy to treat borderline personality disorder, which usually presents with unstable self-image, unstable moods, and impulsivity. Psychoanalysts address underlying personality rather than symptoms, so personality disorders are their bailiwick. Psychoanalytic approaches identify and change the instability, maladaptive behaviors, and ego of the concerned person (Bradley & Westen, 2005). The psychoanalyst aims to understand the individual's childhood years and their relationships with their parents and other family members. This knowledge helps the therapist rectify specific childhood events that influenced that individual's personality development and helps correlate the present beliefs to realize the split personalities, thereby modifying their ability to regulate their emotions (Bradley & Westen, 2005). Some studies also suggest that psychodynamic psychotherapy is highly effective for various personality disorders (Gabbard, 2000; Leichsenring & Leibing, 2003). Furthermore, Abbass et al. (2011) found that psychodynamic psychotherapy is most effective if personality disorder accompanies depression.

6.3.4 Family Systems Therapy

Family systems therapy is a multidisciplinary therapeutic approach that believes in a social context in which humans live and focuses on the dynamic relationships in a particular system. Family systems therapy is grounded on the concept that considers family as an emotional unit and individuals cannot be separated from their relationship network. This approach is associated with every individual's desires, needs, thoughts, and behaviors within a system and impacts others. Any alteration in the interrelationship between individuals affects the whole family system. The therapy aims to recognize the need for change in a specific family system. Interventions first focus on processing first-order change that modifies behavior without significant change in the system's structure and functional patterns. Next, it aims to process for second-order change to modify the structure of its members' system and functional patterns to build an improved system (Segal et al., 2011). The therapist ought to employ a common ground strategy instead of reproaching one individual as the primary source of increasing calamity. The whole process should emphasize that perhaps all the involved parties can improve communication between them.

Family systems therapy aims to fix the system's structure by breaking the existing interrelationships in a family (Segal et al., 2011). Family systems therapy approaches every part of the system. This approach's major strength is that the therapy does not fully focus on the individual who needs to be changed; instead, it evaluates the whole system of interrelated relationships to create a modified system. Moreover, the system reveals people's complexities and their interactions with others that lead to an array of behaviors, thoughts, and beliefs in a broader perspective. This is considered another strength as it integrates fundamental ideas into our society (Segal et al., 2011). However, some weaknesses limit the applicability of this approach. First, although this therapy recognizes issues of past relationships, it only emphasizes the current relationships in a system (Segal et al., 2011). Also, measuring the exact alterations within a system is difficult due to existing multiple systems and how they took place over time. Moreover, this approach only explores the system, not the individual. Therefore, this model does not investigate any individual problem, even if it needs to be evaluated (Segal et al., 2011). It is also confusing how the system theory works in circumstances when we know that care approaches should be individualized because many layers from an individual's history, culture, and environment and their changes are challenging to measure.

6.3.4.1   Family/Systems Therapy for Depression

Family systems therapy is considered useful in treating older adults and their family members, especially while caring for chronic diseases (Segal et al., 2011). This approach allows different people to be included, which may affect the outcomes. Caregiving can be considered a social context, and alterations in roles in the caregiver and care recipient relationships may disrupt the entire family system's functioning. These alterations further aggravate when various stressors and unsatisfactory support from other family members come into play, leading to caregiver burden and subsequent depression. The caregiver's depression may influence the other members within the system, ultimately resulting in the patient's institutionalization. Family therapy approaches should be directed to alleviate the caregiver's burden to reduce various risks associated with it. In a randomized controlled trial, Eisdorfer et al. (2003) found that depressed caregivers of persons with dementia experienced a significant reduction in depressive symptoms 6 months after receiving structural ecosystem therapy added with computer-based technology support from family and other social supports.

6.3.4.2   Family/Systems Therapy for Anxiety and Other Phobias

Family systems therapy is also used to treat older adults with anxiety disorders. Generalized anxiety disorder is found to be linked with interpersonal difficulties such as relationship distress. Relationship distress is precipitated by family abuse and violence, as well as poor interrelationships, such as cutting people off from another person, due to poor anxiety management (Whisman, 2007). Spousal caregiving often requires meeting dependent partner's functional limitations for codependency. This necessity may create relationship distress and subsequent anxiety. Therefore, family systems strategies should focus on second-order changes to alter functioning and increase independence.

6.3.4.3   Family/Systems Therapy for Personality Disorders

Family therapy is also used to manage personality disorders, particularly when the concerned person is in a relationship or living within a family (Beck et al., 2015). This treatment approach helps individuals with personality disorders identify relevant negative thoughts and interpersonal beliefs. Family therapy may also support the concerned person to modify maladaptive behavior. Individuals with a personality disorder might isolate themselves instead of expressing thoughts if their family has unsatisfactory interpersonal communication and fear that interpersonal sharing may create conflict. Family therapy must aim to build a relationship between the patent, family, and professionals (Segal et al., 2011).

6.4   Conclusion

Although it was not surprising to see that older adults in the United States have a low rate of receiving mental health services, it was surprising to learn that the causes are more or less the same as what was found in India. Therefore, at least regarding the outcome, the scenario of a so-called developed country is the same as that of a so-called developing one. This is probably because of the identical universal mentality of both the caregivers' and the care receivers' perspectives, which could not be mitigated even by workforce and infrastructure development. At the same time, it can be assumed that as the population ages, more older adults would like to use these services because they are growing into the culture of accepting mental illness, along with a general understanding of what it is. It has been estimated that in the United States, we will need 5000 geropsychologists by 2020; currently, we have nearly 700 only (Molinari, 2020b). Current research suggests that older adults do not have as many functional, psychological problems as their younger counterparts; attachment styles remain relatively consistent with the progression of age and are often relevant to caregiving status, coping styles, and day-to-day stressors (Molinari, 2020b). Therefore, the culture change of accepting mental illness needs a mass-awareness program, and certainly the initiative should come from the government level in any country.

We only know the tip of the iceberg regarding the management of mental health problems. The impacts of globalization have made human life more constrained. The reduction in executive functioning might be a normal part of aging, which has implications regarding independent living for older adults at advanced ages. If late-onset depression and anxiety are related to age-related changes in cognitive functioning, perhaps older adults need more support than has been thought for things such as financial decision-making (V. Molinari, personal communication, October 31, 2020). The gradual "extinction" of the extended multigenerational family has provided us a lifestyle full of loneliness, boredom, and helplessness; we are pretending our happy presence in social media, struggling in a stifling condition. Stress has engulfed our life; we do not know the way out. Formal caregivers are only trying to provide their care from theoretical knowledge; however, they are also encapsulated in a world of stress.

Concerning the earlier discussion, it should be an obvious question whether various therapies for mental illnesses are truly effective in their capacity. Are we applying those purposefully or just as a mechanical professional tool? For a country or community where the clinician-patient ratio is higher, it may be effective, but where the same proportion is lower than average, how could we manage those patients? Is not the management of mental disorders a luxury in countries with low socioeconomic status? Is not treating older adults' mental disorders a waste of time in a country with an enormous population? This is not just raising questions about the efficacy of the therapy procedures; instead, it also points to the way it is delivered. Is there any chance to cure? Is there any intention of the therapist to cure their client in the era of medicalization? One of the "good" things about the COVID-19 pandemic in US healthcare is that the government has been paying for telemedicine, reducing expenses, and reaching poor rural folks (V. Molinari, personal communication, October 8, 2020). Otherwise, we are moving toward a black hole.

Finally, it would be a good idea to relate mental health issues with the Baltes idea of wisdom, i.e., "all old people are not wise, and not all wise people are older" (Molinari, 2020b). When we report the demographic picture of a study, we often report formal education as an important variable. Why is that? Is it pragmatic? Why do we overemphasize formal education in our thinking about wisdom? Is it only because most scholars discussing wisdom have formal education and may believe they have the best chance to be wise? Or are we formally representing a formal education system just to achieve our formal milestones (maybe a degree/promotion/grant!)? The recent research on resilience strikes a balance here, however, and researchers now realize that wisdom can be generated from some challenging non-academic life experiences. A 10-year-old boy/girl in a low-economic-level country, where child labor is a norm, may become wiser due to his/her life struggles than even an older adult and so-called educated person of a different environment. How could we explain that?

References

Abbass, A., Town, J., & Driessen, E. (2011). The efficacy of short-term psychodynamic psychotherapy for depressive disorders with comorbid personality disorder. *Psychiatry, 74*(1), 58–71. https://doi.org/10.1521/psyc.2011.74.1.58

Ayers, C. R., Strickland, K., & Wetherell, J. L. (2015). Evidence-based treatment for late-life generalized anxiety disorder. In P. A. Areán (Ed.), *Treatment of late-life depression, anxiety, trauma, and substance abuse*. American Psychological Association.

Bankar, M. A., Chaudhari, S. K., & Chaudhari, K. D. (2013). Impact of long-term Yoga practice on sleep quality and quality of life in the elderly. *Journal of Ayurveda and Integrative Medicine, 4*(1), 28–32. https://doi.org/10.4103/0975-9476.109548

Beck, A. T., Davis, D. D., & Freeman, A. (2015). *Cognitive therapy of personality disorders*. Third edition. New York: Guilford Publications.

Beekman, A. T., Deeg, D. J., van Tilburg, T., Smit, J. H., Hooijer, C., & van Tilburg, W. (1995). Major and minor depression in later life: a study of prevalence and risk factors. *Journal of Affective Disorders, 36*(1-2), 65–75. https://doi.org/10.1016/0165-0327(95)00061-5

Bhattacharyya, K. K., Hueluer, G., Meng, H., & Hyer, K. (2020). Mind-body practices in U.S. adults: Prevalence and correlates. *Complementary Therapies in Medicine, 52*, 102501. https://doi.org/10.1016/j.ctim.2020.102501

Bisson, J. I., Cosgrove, S., Lewis, C., & Robert, N. P. (2015). Post-traumatic stress disorder. *BMJ (Clinical Research Ed.), 351*, h6161. https://doi.org/10.1136/bmj.h6161

Bleichmar, H. B. (1996). Some subtypes of depression and their implications for psychoanalytic treatment. *The International Journal of Psychoanalysis, 77*(Pt 5), 935–961.

Boag, S. (2014). Ego, drives, and the dynamics of internal objects. *Frontiers in Psychology, 5*, 666. https://doi.org/10.3389/fpsyg.2014.00666

Bonnín, C., Reinares, M., Martínez-Arán, A., Jiménez, E., Sánchez-Moreno, J., Solé, B., Montejo, L., & Vieta, E. (2019). Improving functioning, quality of life, and well-being in patients with bipolar disorder. *The International Journal of Neuropsychopharmacology, 22*(8), 467–477. https://doi.org/10.1093/ijnp/pyz018

Bradley, R., & Westen, D. (2005). The psychodynamics of borderline personality disorder: A view from developmental psychopathology. *Development and Psychopathology, 17*(04), 927–957. https://doi.org/10.1017/s0954579405050443

Burgio, L. D., & Burgio, K. L. (1986). Behavioral gerontology: Application of behavioral methods to the problems of older adults. *Journal of Applied Behavior Analysis, 19*(4), 321–328. https://doi.org/10.1901/jaba.1986.19-321

Compton, M. T., Kelley, M. E., Pope, A., Smith, K., Broussard, B., Reed, T. A., DiPolito, J. A., Druss, B. G., Li, C., & Lott Haynes, N. (2016). Opening doors to recovery: Recidivism and recovery among persons with serious mental illnesses and repeated hospitalizations. *Psychiatric Services (Washington, D.C.), 67*(2), 169–175. https://doi.org/10.1176/appi.ps.201300482

Desai, A. K., Seraji, M., Redden, M., & Tatini, R. (2010). Schizophrenia in older adults how to adjust treatment to address aging patients' changing symptoms, comorbidities. *Current Psychiatry, 9*(9), 23–28.

Driessen, E., & Hollon, S. D. (2010). Cognitive behavioral therapy for mood disorders: efficacy, moderators and mediators. *The Psychiatric Clinics of North America, 33*(3), 537–555. https://doi.org/10.1016/j.psc.2010.04.005

Eisdorfer, C., Czaja, S. J., Loewenstein, D. A., Rubert, M. P., Argüelles, S., Mitrani, V. B., & Szapocznik, J. (2003). The effect of a family therapy and technology-based intervention on caregiver depression. *The Gerontologist, 43*(4), 521–531. https://doi.org/10.1093/geront/43.4.521

Ekselius, L. (2018). Personality disorder: a disease in disguise. *Upsala Journal of Medical Sciences, 123*(4), 194–204. https://doi.org/10.1080/03009734.2018.1526235

Gabbard, G. O. (2000). Psychotherapy of personality disorders. *The Journal of Psychotherapy Practice and Research, 9*(1), 1–6.

Gale, C., & Davidson, O. (2007). Generalised anxiety disorder. *BMJ (Clinical Research Ed.), 334*(7593), 579–581. https://doi.org/10.1136/bmj.39133.559282.BE

Garcia, R. (2017). Neurobiology of fear and specific phobias. *Learning & Memory (Cold Spring Harbor, N.Y.), 24*(9), 462–471. https://doi.org/10.1101/lm.044115.116

Gholipour, A., Abolghasemi, S. h., Gholinia, K., & Taheri, S. (2012). Token reinforcement therapeutic approach is more effective than exercise for controlling negative symptoms of schizophrenic patients: A randomized controlled trial. *International Journal of Preventive Medicine, 3*(7), 466–470.

Gum, A. M., Iser, L., & Petkus, A. (2010). Behavioral health service utilization and preferences of older adults receiving home-based aging services. *The American journal of Geriatric Psychiatry, 18*(6), 491–501. https://doi.org/10.1097/JGP.0b013e3181c29495

Granholm, E., McQuaid, J. R., McClure, F. S., Auslander, L. A., Perivoliotis, D., Pedrelli, P., Patterson, T., & Jeste, D. V. (2005). A randomized, controlled trial of cognitive behavioral social skills training for middle-aged and older outpatients with chronic schizophrenia. *The American Journal of Psychiatry, 162*(3), 520–529. https://doi.org/10.1176/appi.ajp.162.3.520

Hans, E., & Hiller, W. (2013). A meta-analysis of nonrandomized effectiveness studies on outpatient cognitive behavioral therapy for adult anxiety disorders. *Clinical Psychology Review, 33*(8), 954–964. https://doi.org/10.1016/j.cpr.2013.07.003

Hofmann, S. G., Asnaani, A., Vonk, I. J., Sawyer, A. T., & Fang, A. (2012). The efficacy of cognitive behavioral therapy: A review of meta-analyses. *Cognitive Therapy and Research, 36*(5), 427–440. https://doi.org/10.1007/s10608-012-9476-1

Kaczkurkin, A. N., & Foa, E. B. (2015). Cognitive-behavioral therapy for anxiety disorders: an update on the empirical evidence. *Dialogues in Clinical Neuroscience, 17*(3), 337–346.

Kanter, J. W., Busch, A. M., Weeks, C. E., & Landes, S. J. (2008). The nature of clinical depression: symptoms, syndromes, and behavior analysis. *The Behavior Analyst, 31*(1), 1–21. https://doi.org/10.1007/BF03392158

Kaiser, A. M., Cook, J. M., Glick, D. M., & Moye, J. (2019). Posttraumatic Stress Disorder in Older Adults: A Conceptual Review. *Clinical Gerontologist, 42*(4), 359–376. https://doi.org/1 0.1080/07317115.2018.1539801

Lack, C. W. (2012). Obsessive-compulsive disorder: Evidence-based treatments and future directions for research. *World Journal of Psychiatry, 2*(6), 86–90. https://doi.org/10.5498/wjp. v2.i6.86

Leichsenring, F., & Leibing, E. (2003). The effectiveness of psychodynamic therapy and cognitive behavior therapy in the treatment of personality disorders: A meta-analysis. *American Journal of Psychiatry, 160*(7), 1223–232. https://doi.org/10.1176/appi.ajp.160.7.1223.

Lewinsohn, P. M. (1975). The behavioral study and treatment of depression. In M. Hersen, R. M. Eisler, & P. M. Miller (Eds.), *Progress in behavioral modification* (Vol. 1, pp. 331–359). Academic.

Livingston, J. D., & Boyd, J. E. (2010). Correlates and consequences of internalized stigma for people living with mental illness: A systematic review and meta-analysis. *Social Science & Medicine (1982), 71*(12), 2150–2161. https://doi.org/10.1016/j.socscimed.2010.09.030

Mai, E., & Buysse, D. J. (2008). Insomnia: Prevalence, impact, pathogenesis, differential diagnosis, and evaluation. *Sleep Medicine Clinics, 3*(2), 167–174. https://doi.org/10.1016/j. jsmc.2008.02.001

Malmberg, L., & Fenton, M. (2001). Individual psychodynamic psychotherapy and psychoanalysis for schizophrenia and severe mental illness. *The Cochrane Database of Systematic Reviews, 3*, CD001360. https://doi.org/10.1002/14651858.CD001360

Matusiewicz, A. K., Hopwood, C. J., Banducci, A. N., & Lejuez, C. W. (2010). The effectiveness of cognitive behavioral therapy for personality disorders. *The Psychiatric Clinics of North America, 33*(3), 657–685. https://doi.org/10.1016/j.psc.2010.04.007

McLeod, S. A. (2019). *Id, ego, and superego.* Simply Psychology. Retrieved from: https://www. simplypsychology.org/psyche.html

Miller, E. A., & Rosenheck, R. A. (2006). Risk of nursing home admission in association with mental illness nationally in the Department of Veterans Affairs. *Medical Care, 44*(4), 343–351. https://doi.org/10.1097/01.mlr.0000204008.83633.ed

Miloyan, B., Byrne, G. J., & Pachana, N. A. (2014). Late-life anxiety. In N. A. Pachana & K. Laidlaw (Eds.), *The Oxford handbook of clinical geropsychology* (pp. 470–489). Oxford University Press.

Mitchell, A. J., Chan, M., Bhatti, H., Halton, M., Grassi, L., Johansen, C., & Meader, N. (2011). Prevalence of depression, anxiety, and adjustment disorder in oncological, haematological, and palliative-care settings: a meta-analysis of 94 interview-based studies. *The Lancet. Oncology, 12*(2), 160–174. https://doi.org/10.1016/S1470-2045(11)70002-X

Molinari, V. (Producer). (2020a, November 4). *Serious mental illness in older adults.* [PowerPoint slides].

Molinari, V. (Producer). (2020b, September 23). *Psychoanalysis and aging.* [PowerPoint slides].

Molinari, V., Kier, F. J., & Rosowsky, E. (2006). SOC, personality, and long-term care. In L. Hyer & R. C. Intrieri (Eds.), *Geropsychological interventions in long-term care* (pp. 139–155). Springer.

Patel, K. R., Cherian, J., Gohil, K., & Atkinson, D. (2014). Schizophrenia: Overview and treatment options. *P & T: A Peer-Reviewed Journal for Formulary Management, 39*(9), 638–645.

Petkus, A. J., & Wetherell, J. L. (2013). Acceptance and commitment therapy with older adults: Rationale and considerations. *Cognitive and Behavioral Practice, 20*(1), 47–56. https://doi. org/10.1016/j.cbpra.2011.07.004

Power, G. A. (2010). *Dementia beyond drugs: Changing the culture of care.* Health professional Press (ISBN 978-1-932529-56-2).

Ridenour, J. M. (2016). Psychodynamic model and treatment of schizotypal personality disorder. *Psychoanalytic Psychology, 33*(1), 129–146.

Reynolds, K., Pietrzak, R. H., El-Gabalawy, R., Mackenzie, C. S., & Sareen, J. (2015). Prevalence of psychiatric disorders in U.S. older adults: Findings from a nationally representative survey. *World Psychiatry, 14*(1), 74–81. https://doi.org/10.1002/wps.20193

Robbins, M. (2012). The successful psychoanalytic therapy of a schizophrenic woman. *Psychodynamic Psychiatry, 40*(4), 575–608. https://doi.org/10.1521/pdps.2012.40.4.575

Rudaz, M., Ledermann, T., Margraf, J., Becker, E. S., & Craske, M. G. (2017). The moderating role of avoidance behavior on anxiety over time: Is there a difference between social anxiety disorder and specific phobia? *PloS one, 12*(7), e0180298. https://doi.org/10.1371/journal.pone.0180298

Ruscio, A. M., Stein, D. J., Chiu, W. T., & Kessler, R. C. (2010). The epidemiology of obsessive-compulsive disorder in the National Comorbidity Survey Replication. *Molecular psychiatry, 15*(1), 53–63. https://doi.org/10.1038/mp.2008.94

Segal, D. L., Qualls, S. H., & Smyer, M. A. (2011). *Aging and Mental Health* (3rd ed.). Wiley-Blackwell.

Scogin, F. R., Welsh, D., Hanson, A., Stump, J., & Coates, A. (2005). Evidence-based psychotherapies for depression in older adults. *Clinical Psychology: Science and Practice, 12*, 222–237. https://doi.org/10.1093/clipsy/bpi033

Sindi, S., Kåreholt, I., Johansson, L., Skoog, J., Sjöberg, L., Wang, H. X., Johansson, B., Fratiglioni, L., Soininen, H., Solomon, A., Skoog, I., & Kivipelto, M. (2018). Sleep disturbances and dementia risk: A multicenter study. *Alzheimer's and Dementia, 14*(10), 1235–1242. https://doi.org/10.1016/j.jalz.2018.05.012

Troxel, W. M., Buysse, D. J., Matthews, K. A., Kip, K. E., Strollo, P. J., Hall, M., Drumheller, O., & Reis, S. E. (2010). Sleep symptoms predict the development of the metabolic syndrome. *Sleep, 33*(12), 1633–1640. https://doi.org/10.1093/sleep/33.12.1633

Wang, P. S., Berglund, P., Olfson, M., Pincus, H. A., Wells, K. B., & Kessler, R. C. (2005). Failure and delay in initial treatment contact after first onset of mental disorders in the National Comorbidity Survey Replication. *Archives of General Psychiatry, 62*(6), 603–613. https://doi.org/10.1001/archpsyc.62.6.603

Wang, J., Wu, X., Lai, W., Long, E., Zhang, X., Li, W., Zhu, Y., Chen, C., Zhong, X., Liu, Z., Wang, D., & Lin, H. (2017). Prevalence of depression and depressive symptoms among outpatients: a systematic review and meta-analysis. *BMJ Open, 7*(8), e017173. https://doi.org/10.1136/bmjopen-2017-017173

Whisman, M. A. (2007). Marital distress and DSM-IV psychiatric disorders in a population-based national survey. *Journal of Abnormal Psychology, 116*(3), 638–643. https://doi.org/10.1037/0021-843X.116.3.638

Wolitzky-Taylor, K. B., Horowitz, J. D., Powers, M. B., & Telch, M. J. (2008). Psychological approaches in the treatment of specific phobias: A meta-analysis. *Clinical Psychology Review, 28*(6), 1021–1037. https://doi.org/10.1016/j.cpr.2008.02.007

Chapter 7
Aging and Dementia

7.1 Cognitive Health and Its Impairment

7.1.1 Prevalence

"Brain death" is considered the demarcation line between whether a person is alive or not, and this proves the significance of the brain in our life. The human brain is a complex organ, both in its anatomical structure and physiological functioning. The brain is responsible for nearly all motor and sensory functions in our body. Memory is one of the vital functions of the human brain, which involves "encoding, retention, and retrieval of information and experiences" (Hoyer & Verhaeghen, 2006).

Aging is an unavoidable part of the normal life course of every human being. In the last century, the average human life span increased by about 30 years. As we pass through an era of a demographic shift, we now have millions of older citizens. As we grow older, our knowledge grows, our experience grows, but at the same time, we lose so many things with our progression toward elderhood. Our general cognitive abilities tend to decline throughout adulthood. Dementia, which is considered progressive deterioration of the cognitive function of an individual, is one of the most unrecognized and undertreated chronic conditions in the present world (Mantri et al., 2019). As the older adult population is aging globally, the number of persons with cognitive decline and dementia is increasing in every part of the world, including India. It is presumed that the total number of persons with dementia (PWD) will double nearly every 20 years, increasing from 46.8 million in 2015 to 131.5 million in 2050 (Alzheimer's Disease International, 2015).

Advancements in diagnosis and treatment protocol have resulted in increased longevity of human life. However, as the non-identification of dementia is much more common, the definitive treatment for the majority of dementia is still unavailable. Often, common people, even the primary care doctors, ignore the early signs and symptoms of dementia, as they confuse these with normal old-age-related

© The Author(s), under exclusive license to Springer Nature Switzerland AG 2021   81
K. K. Bhattacharyya, *Rethinking the Aging Transition*,
https://doi.org/10.1007/978-3-030-88870-1_7

behaviors. Therefore, the status of dementia persists as the "tip of the iceberg" in present societies, which is more prevalent in the developing countries where the population is humongous. At the country level, the countries were home to over a million people with dementia in 2015; the United States (4.2 million) holds the 2nd spot and India (4.1 million) the 3rd spot behind China (9.5 million) (Alzheimer's Disease International, 2015). In India, only one in ten gets a diagnosis, treatment, and care (Alzheimer's Disease International, 2015). In India, the calculated total societal cost of dementia was estimated to be 3.4 billion USD (INR 147 billion), where nearly 29% of the total cost is the direct medical cost (INR 46.8 billion) (Alzheimer's and Related Disorder Society of India [ARDSI], 2010). Studies suggest that in the other part of the globe, in the United States, total payments in 2015 for all individuals with Alzheimer's disease and other dementia are estimated at 226 billion USD (Alzheimer's Association, 2015). Therefore, it is a global problem, in the truest sense of the term.

7.1.2   Causative Factors

Cognitive health is an essential component of brain health that includes the ability to think, learn, and remember clearly. Although lifestyle factors such as taking care of physical health, healthy dietary habits, social connection, and physical activities are important to maintain good cognitive health, keeping one's mind and body active through cognitive training is considered equally important. Our brain can adapt and develop new abilities throughout our lifetime but show variance. This ability to reorganize and create new ways to develop cognitive functions is called neuroplasticity. The neurocognitive status of the brain does not always reveal memory declination with aging but sometimes results in preservation, even improvement. This complex relationship largely depends on the area of the brain concerned. If we consider working memory, its functions show a large decline with age progression as these are controlled by the prefrontal cortex. In contrast, episodic memory shows less reduction in functioning as this is largely mediated by the hippocampus (Lustig & Lin, 2016). However, semantic memory function shows no such reduction, even sometimes improved functioning, as it is mediated by the anterior temporal lobes. When we consider automatic processing, older persons perform memory tasks like younger ones. When it shows a decline, the condition indicates impending dementia, though the older adults develop partial compensatory functioning as well as compensatory environmental support.

Mild cognitive impairment often precedes dementia, where the cognitive decline, particularly memory decline, exceeds the expected age-related deterioration and usually does not interfere with one's daily ability to function independently (Knopman & Petersen, 2014). On the other hand, dementia, even in its early stages, signals some distinct inability to function independently, with progressive cognitive and behavioral changes (Knopman & Petersen, 2014). Dementia can be classified as primary and secondary. According to disease progression, it is also commonly categorized as reversible or irreversible. In the reversible type, symptoms may be caused by one or more medical conditions that can be treated. These may be drug-induced, vitamin B1 deficiencies, alcohol abuse, depression, and brain tumors, which can cause neurological deficits that resemble dementia. Most of these cases respond to treatment. However, in many other dementia-causing diseases, the damage done to the brain by the disease cannot be reversed, and this is called "primary dementia." Among these diseases—Alzheimer's disease, post-cerebrovascular accident (vascular dementia), Parkinson's disease, Lewy-body dementia, Huntington's disease—frontotemporal lobar degeneration is commonly seen (Saxon et al., 2015). Alzheimer's disease is the most common cause of dementia, which is presently the 6th leading cause of death in the United States (Alzheimer's Association, 2017; Taylor et al., 2017). Alzheimer's disease is a slow progressive neurodegenerative disorder, characterized by memory loss due to neuronal damage in the brain. With the progression of time, the patient cannot even recognize their close family members. Alzheimer's disease has no definite curative intervention available to date. The deposition of amyloid plaques in the gray matter of the brain is the causative factor of this disease.

7.1.3   Predisposing Factors

Although we have a better understanding of the various causes of cognitive impairments, little is known about the predisposing factors responsible for these conditions. Brewster and colleagues discussed different life course events and expectations and demographic impact on cognitive abilities in older adults (Brewster et al., 2014). Their longitudinal study examined 333 older adults who were different regarding their educational, ethnicity, and cognitive backgrounds. They examined how different parameters of an individual's life like childhood socioeconomic status, age, literacy level, physical growth parameters (such as head circumference, knee height), and age-specific recreational activities influence cognition and their relationship with respect to apolipoprotein E and other demographic variables such as ethnicity and language. The authors concluded that those parameters of the life course (like literacy level) were strongly related to individuals' basic cognitive abilities, and those changes were best expressed by age, apolipoprotein E, literacy, and recreational activities of the current age. In my opinion, there are a few gaps present in the study. Though the samples were heterogeneous regarding demographic and cognition standards, the follow-up period was only 4 years (average); cognitive deterioration may take much more time to be fully understood. Also, the study was performed in a smaller geographical location (a portion of Northern California), where the participants lead more or less an equal lifestyle (though the participants' ethnicities were different), so there is a question of international acceptance of the conclusion of the study. Lastly, the parameters included in this study might not contribute to the ultimate difference. In this regard, India is my home country, where there are multiple languages, multiple religions, and multiple ethnicities that coexist in a variety of geographical locations and have different socioeconomic statuses. It would not be an overexaggeration to explore the significance of this study from India's perspective regarding the variables like literacy, language, morphometrics, childhood socioeconomic conditions, apoE, and physical and recreational activities.

Mood disorders in older adults range from subsyndromal depression to bipolar disorders of different intensities (Barry & Byers, 2016). There is also an interrelation that exists between chronic physical diseases and depression. These contribute to the development of dementia in later life, through different internal mechanisms like ischemic structural brain changes, through the hypothalamic-pituitary-adrenal axis, and by alteration of steroid levels. On the other hand, late-life anxiety disorders are found to be as high or even higher in number. These may coexist in high prevalence, which may be influenced by genetic factors, chronic physical diseases, and lifestyle, even family life or marital status such as unmarried or divorced. All of these are greatly affected by psychological factors like spousal bereavement and social support in the form of emotional (like sympathy) and instrumental (like assistance) support. Most of the patients with mental disorders do not feel comfortable discussing their personal problems; they present their physical problems to their physicians but are unaware of the significance of their psychological problems. It is a big challenge for physicians to improve awareness, screening, and prevention processes to detect untreated mental disorders. I can well remember one of my close friends, Mr. Madan Gopal Nath (name changed), who had bipolar disorder. In his late 50s, he had developed alternate episodes of anxiety and depression. Though he had few other comorbidities like hypertension, diabetes (type 2), ischemic heart disease, and benign prostatic hypertrophy, still during the times when he was free of mental abnormalities, he was a very gentle and kind person. However, when the symptoms of mood disorder started, it was tough for his wife to control him. In successive few years, he was compelled to take voluntary retirement from his government job, which caused the development of further depression. In consequence, these aggravated his physical disorders, and he passed away in his mid-60s, leaving his family on a battlefield of struggle.

7.2   Dementia: Does Terminology Matter?

Unlike many other diseases, persons with dementia require support from others, which may come from family members (informal caregiver), paid (formal) caregivers, or different healthcare personnel like doctors, nurses, or other paramedical professionals. Lin and Lewis discussed different terminologies associated with dementia care (2015), to prepare us to be engaged in care works for the massive number of dementia patients. Also, for the upcoming dementia crisis, first, we need to be accustomed to these terminologies. "Dementia-friendly" is the approach taken by the European Union countries, and "dementia capable" is the approach carried out in the United States. The approaches are different in their focus, but the ultimate purpose of both is to provide help for persons with dementia and their families. These are to ensure that these people can live with dignity and can access treatment, care, and support when needed. Another term is "dementia positive," which is the actual involvement of society with dementia patients. The persons with dementia expect from society not only theoretical supports but also to accept their disability; thereby, they can actively live a meaningful life. This article is a vivid presentation of the present scenario and future planning of dementia care. In my opinion, the authors are quite successful in their intention by way of presentation. They expressed hope for a future world where there will be effective dementia treatment and preventive measures. Also, there will be interventions to promote the social involvement of dementia patients and their families, as well as enough scope for social science and biomedical research in this field. Recently another term gaining importance is "dementia inclusive," as if persons with dementia need to be included in our society, avoiding all stigmatization. Some social scientists even want to discard the term "dementia" and raise their hands for only "inclusive." They want to change the term "dementia-friendly communities" to "inclusive and accessible communities." But the inclusion of what and where? What are we concerned about? HIV? Cancer? Tuberculosis? Autism? Or dementia? Which one will be *included*? So, an "inclusive community" is a misnomer like *humanity without a man*. In my opinion, we may consider "dementia inclusive," but anything without the term *dementia* should not be acceptable.

According to the dictionary, *dementia* is a medical condition comprising a group of cognitive and social symptoms that interfere with daily functioning. *Dementia*, being an umbrella term, covers various cognitive impairment and neurodegenerations, causing various functional and behavioral problems manifested by a decline in mental ability severe enough to interfere with daily life. Memory loss is an example. Alzheimer's disease is the most common type of dementia, but it is only a variety; it cannot be used as an umbrella term. The word *dementia* was developed in the late eighteenth century from Latin, "demens," meaning dement or "out of one's mind." In common usage, "dementia" is one of the 10,000 most commonly used words in the Collins dictionary. We cannot avoid the word *dementia* anymore. Still, it is only a word. It is described differently in different languages [American English, dementia; Bengali, smritibhransh; Brazilian Portuguese, demência; Chinese, chīdāi; European Spanish, demencia; French, démence; German, demenz; Hindi, paagalapan; Italian, demenza; Japanese, ninshishō; Korean, baegchi; European Portuguese, demência; Russian, deméncija; Spanish, demencia; Arabic, marad eaqliun; Tamil, mutumai]. Therefore, why should we fight only for a *word*? We should fight against the horrible conditions caused by the problem, irrespective of terminology. We must fight against both the stigma and real dementia, whether friendly or unfriendly, for our protection, to achieve better aging (or aging well), whatever the terminologies are.

In reality, dementia patients are a burden for their family members. In India, there is no "significant" social welfare program currently available that is beneficial to this group of people; "those" available are being engulfed by corruption. The good words are only present theoretically in different academic articles, which give researchers an excellent career opportunity but least benefit the persons with dementia. There are people of different cultures, religions, and socioeconomic statuses in India, but the common fact is the declining attention toward elderlies everywhere.

We should be honest in our life course whatever our profession may be—toward our work, toward our morality, and toward our social duties. We, each and every one of us, need to change our attitude and focus; otherwise, we are not able to extend our hand toward our older generation. We should be loyal to our ethics and honesty. Because of being a medical doctor, I always feel some extra responsibilities for these people.

7.3   Dementia: A Case Study from a Caregiver's Perspective

At this point of discussion, I want to mention one person who is not only related to the topic of discussion but also one of the most influential persons for my career change. She is my maternal grandmother, the late Mrs. Bimala Bhattacharyya. I grew up with my grandmother, who greatly influenced my values and thoughts. Because of her kindness toward me, I have a deep respect for her and older adults in general. My grandmother suffered from Alzheimer's disease, as diagnosed by a neuropsychiatrist by the method of exclusion. She had a huge disability in her late 70s, although she was otherwise fit and free from any chronic physical diseases. She was very disciplined in life, educated, and a homemaker but was on regular physical and mental activities and had no addiction. My grandparents maintained their married relationship in a compensatory and optimal way. They enjoyed their whole life within their extended family, having good health (both physical and mental), well-being (spiritual and both intra- and interrelationship with others), and even during their late-life cognitive impairments. However, after hearing the news of the sudden passing away of my grandfather, my grandmother became severely ill, and within the next 24 h, she forgot everything about her current days. Within a very short period, she literally lost every meaning in life (maybe due to the loss of compensatory relationship) and a few months later left us. Alzheimer's disease is usually a slower onset disorder; however, I came across a rapid deterioration in this case.

On the other hand, the situation of my mother, Mrs. Gita Bhattacharyya, is different. She has multiple comorbidities and, along with her formal and informal caregivers, endured a tough and confusing time. She is in her late 60s and suffering from dementia (most probably Alzheimer's disease by symptoms), chronic colitis, obsessive-compulsive disorder, osteoarthritis (seronegative), and many other age-related health problems. Her primary health problems are not due to old age but aggravated by old age. She is a homemaker but not leading a sedentary lifestyle. She lives in a three-storied building with my father (who is also in his late 60s). She was very energetic till a few months back and had done a lot of hard work since her younger days. She had no diseases as such, except obsessive-compulsive disorder and colitis, until her early 60s. The obsessive-compulsive disorder took all her energy during that time; she felt the motivation to clean everything like an addiction. Gradually she developed postural hypotension and mixed anxiety-depression disorder, and dementia developed over time. As a physician, it was surprising to see how even dementia could not be able to remove behaviors of obsessive-compulsive disorder from her mind. Knowingly or unknowingly, I became a member of the team engaged in her "person-centered" care. I, along with a neuropsychiatrist, a homeopathy physician, my father, sister, and my mother herself, all worked together on her deteriorating health condition. We jotted down some health prevention measures for her. However, one challenge that we faced in every step of management was the ego problem between generations.

First, as she moves everywhere in a three-storied building, it was proposed to create a guard/handrail in the staircases to prevent falls (and associated bony injuries) as a primary preventive measure. This step was a measure for identifying and targeting risk factors for her to prevent disease before it starts. Second, it was proposed to shift her residence to her son's house, where she can avail herself of the restrooms on every floor, to avoid stairs as much as possible. As she has obsessive-compulsive disorder and associated colitis, there is an increased chance of falls on the slippery floors in our old house. Persons with dementia often lose their balance; therefore, the risk factors for falls and other consequences should be the primary prevention measures that my parents were in denial. Third, it was proposed to make the food habit better as directed by the physician (and nutritionist) to allow for maximal nutritional status. Still, they refused to take homemade meals from their son's/daughter's houses; instead, they depended on takeaway food. It is required for her to take dopaminergic food items, such as turmeric, almond, dark chocolate, blueberries, and banana, that should be incorporated into the daily dietary items to fight against dementia. However, it is impossible to watch every person at their homes all the time. Fourth, it was suggested and emphasized to engage in mind-body therapy, with the practice of yoga and meditation, but my mother was reluctant to do all those, too. Finally, it was suggested to increase social connection and spiritual health as tertiary (also quaternary) level of prevention. Now the experimental social model is considered the only option for dementia management over the traditional medical model. This involvement may be helpful for the obsessive-compulsive disorder as well. After consultation with the neuropsychiatrist, we stopped all the medications prescribed (for dementia) for my mother. Due to severe drowsiness, she fell multiple times on the ground and developed pressure ulcers in the dependent parts (mostly sacral and scapular regions). We managed the primary incidents and stopped all medications as a part of secondary prevention (preventing disease while still asymptomatic or in early stages using screening). This is the alteration from traditional management, and it varies case by case. However, we have continued the other medicines (like those for osteoarthritis). Surprisingly, when her drowsiness disappeared, she became engaged in obsessive-compulsive disorder behaviors. As a physician, I have guided my father not to restrict her, as this is her only movement and activity. The only thing that I am worried about as a physician is her setup at home. We are giving symptomatic treatment, and she is much better now than before. She can do almost every daily activity by herself, though very slowly.

Even after coming to the United States, a so-called developed country, I realized that dementia is more or less similar to that of India; the main difference is that in the United States, the population is smaller and people are more self-sufficient than in India. In my opinion, in India, the persistence of multigenerational extended family culture may be a cause for less self-sufficiency and more dependency in the relationship. The healthcare cost in the United States is much more compared to that of India, where the medical facility is available much more easily but may make it more prone for misuse. In both countries, however, the older adults have a critical need for better support to age well, but everywhere the caregivers are lower in number. In India in 2015, the number of persons with dementia was 116,553 (8.9% of the population aged 60 years or older). It is projected to be 330,043 (19.4% of the population aged 60+ years) in 2050. Whereas in the United States, the number was 66,545 (20.7% of the population aged 60+ years) in 2015. This number may go up to 108,326 (27.9% of the population aged 60+ years) in the year 2050 (United Nations, 2015). In India, the specialized personnel for these groups of persons are very limited in number (only 0.43 for taking care of one million persons with dementia) (ARDSI, 2010); in contrast, in the United States, although the number is much higher, they still are not enough to cover the necessities. In the United States, there are about 15.7 million adult family (informal) caregivers who care for individuals with Alzheimer's disease or other dementia (Alzheimer's Disease International, 2015). Regarding formal care, presently, there are 7,428 certified geriatricians and 1,629 geriatric psychiatrists available in this field (The American Geriatrics Society, 2016). Regarding other human resources, approximately one percent of registered nurses, physician assistants, and pharmacists exist in the field of geriatrics. Only four percent of geriatric-certified social workers have engaged themselves in their formal duties (Institute of Medicine, 2015).

Therefore, we must make the workforce our priority. However, this can happen only when the concerned government pays attention and makes it a priority. They should implement more policies and programs targeting dementia, spread more awareness by advertisements and campaigns in collaboration with different NGOs, take adequate measures to train professionals in this field, and counsel and support families with dementia patients. There should be some internationally accepted collaborative policies involving all the countries of the world.

7.4   The Virtual Dementia Tour

In clinical practice, I always remained cautious about dementia, one of the common under-recognized medical conditions and felt some extra responsibilities for the persons with dementia. Therefore, from a natural desire, after hearing about the "virtual dementia tour" (VDT) (organized by the Second Wind Dreams) for the first time, I have not wasted a single minute to register myself as a candidate there.

From the program literature, it was already clear that the virtual dementia tour (Beville, 2017) was the first of its kind, is clinically proven and evidence-based, and is a proven source of education, resulting in better care for dementia patients. Therefore, I was very much eager to participate in that activity/training program. Being a medical doctor, I expected to get a firsthand experience from this event by identifying the requirements of those living with dementia. I wanted to compare that with what I learned from various readings and clinical experiences to date to apply these experiences in real-life situations and while treating patients with cognitive impairments. Being a volunteer, I got the chance to experience the *virtual dementia tour* firsthand.

After completion of the initial formalities, I entered the garbing room. One of our co-volunteers helped me wear specially designed shoe inserts under the sole (inside the shoes), a pair of plastic gloves, then a pair of thick woolen gloves on my hands. The places for some fingers of the gloves were stitched so that those three fingers could not be moved separately. I had to wear a spectacle, which was designed in such a manner that the vision became restricted. Almost two-fifths of the glass (on lateral sides of both the glasses) was hazy; in the remaining part, there was a circular marking (in each one), through which one can hardly visualize anything because of its high refractive power. Lastly, I had to wear a headset. I have seen "spacesuits" but never had an experience wearing that, yet I do not know why the word first came into my mind after walking the first step with those things on.

After entering the actual *virtual dementia tour* room, the connection of the head-set was on, and I heard only a mixed but "h-i-s-s-ing" sound of moderate intensity. However, it was bothersome and took all my attention. Then someone came in front; I could only identify her as the gentle lady who was one of the organizers, but this was an intuition from our previous setup and would probably be very difficult if someone new came up. She instructed something that I could not follow due to lack of attention (sound of the headset) and visual difficulty. She took me in front of a table, where I saw so many everyday household things. For the first few moments (maybe seconds or minutes), I was wondering about what to do there. Time was running out, and I shouted, "what do I have to do here?" Someone came and repeated something that I could not follow; it was indeed a difficult situation. Under a dimmed light and with a reduced vision, I started to concentrate on the table where everything was laid down in an unorganized manner. A wall clock was there but not working; two pencil batteries were nearby, but I could not fix it because my hands were unable to perform more delicate works of that kind. There was a candle, lighter, cups, and teapots, but I realized those tasks are challenging to perform. Then I saw some towels and picked one up with broad fingers and put that in an organized manner and repeated the task for three consecutive towels and got a little bit of con-fidence. Continuously, however, I was disturbed by the sounds of the headset. Then I picked up a leather belt and put it in an organized manner. There was an uncom-fortable feeling of the fiber pad underneath the foot, and I discovered a few shirts and ties were hanging on a hook nearby, but before moving toward that direction, the sound of a hooter rang loudly, and someone instructed to stop. I first took the headset off because this thing troubled me the most. I came out of the *virtual demen-tia tour* room and engaged again in work as a volunteer, helping others in the train-ing program. The actual picture was clear after attending the debriefing session.

The *virtual dementia tour* experience was scheduled for 8 min only, which I came to know afterward; however, I did not realize that inside the room. Instead, I felt like an examination, where time passed very quickly, and I struggled to do every job. It was only after the debriefing session, and when I had leisure time to recapitulate the experience, that I realized the significance of the program. I reckon 8 min were not enough; it should be a few minutes more, at least for 12–15 min, because for the first few minutes, it was very confusing about what to do or not to do. It was a real, powerful journey to experience the realities of daily life with dementia. It was a sudden realization that now I could not do the tasks that were so simple for me earlier. I could not fix a battery in a wall clock, could not put the button of my shirt in the proper buttonhole, and even could not pour tea from a teapot into a cup, which I had never experienced before. This was mainly because of the inability to move the fingers (especially the thumb, which is why the thumb made the primates superior to other animals) freely or the inability to control other body parts. My self-confidence level had gone down. I do not know how to compare these performances with a person with dementia (because of their cognitive impairment). But I believe strongly that they also can realize their inability to perform their once easily achievable tasks. This is probably the most pathetic sensation of a person with dementia, at least for those having mild to moderate dementia, in front of surrounding people. This inferiority complex may provoke them to withdraw from their surrounding world. As a negative feedback effect, it leads them toward severe dementia. I can relate this situation with one of my once-read characters, Mrs. Alice Hobson (Gawande, 2014). I can well realize her condition regarding withdrawal from the surrounding world after being diagnosed with dementia and forced to go to a safer home, against her will, by her family members. This type of situation is also confusing for their caregivers. In his early 80s, we saw Felix and realized how difficult the job is when caring for his wife, Bella (Gawande, 2014). The life-changing experience in the *virtual dementia tour* has given me the insight and empathy needed to provide better person-centered care by helping me identify personally with the needs of persons with dementia. Dr. Gawande told us about honesty, not only as a doctor but also as a human being in real-life situations. I can well relate this feeling to my personal life. My grandmother was suffering from Alzheimer's disease, and she loved chocolate very much. I only gave her one or two chocolates each time I met her in her later life; however, being a busy professional, I did not have much time to assist in her daily activities.

7.5   The Virtual Dementia Tour: Realizations

However, suddenly, this *virtual dementia tour* has given me a new direction in the form of a new realization. What I am thinking is only one side of the coin. My parents might not feel the same way. Even I do not know now whether my mother can think at all or not. I went inside the almost dark *virtual dementia tour* room, knowing from the outside that it is daytime. However, now I can imagine the condition of persons with dementia who have lost their orientation of time. The glass I wore only allowed a cone-shaped vision (like the vision of a fish from inside out of the water level) due to its lateral part's haziness, and that also can be done only through a high refractive powered circular portion. Due to less flexibility of eyeball muscles, cataracts, corneal haziness, and overall variable sensory deficit, vision becomes restricted in these individuals' real lives. Conductive as well as sensory-neural deafness is also very common to these patients. Due to the stiffness of the tympanic membrane and frequent calcification of the Eustachian tube, a continuous h-i-s-s sound is also monotonous but unavoidable for them. This mechanical sound effect was created in our *virtual dementia tour* experience. Also, there were few other sounds of different pitches. Persons with dementia face massive difficulty concentrating, which is aggravated by the unusual sound produced in our surroundings knowingly or unknowingly, which causes distraction. The associated stress causes sudden acetylcholine secretion, followed by adrenaline secretion, which results in increased heart rate, respiration rate, and blood pressure. This situation was nicely created in the *virtual dementia tour*. The median nerve controls our thumb, index, and middle fingers, and ring and little fingers by the ulnar nerve. Other different small collateral nerves control the fine movements of small muscles of the fingers. This complex process is lost with the sensory-neural deficit in these individuals, so crude movements are only possible. Medial three fingers and lateral two fingers can only move together, but individual finger movement becomes severely restricted, and finer movements (like when we perform tasks by fingertips) are grossly hampered. I experienced this while performing tasks with the gloves (with some fingers stitched) on my hands. There was a pair of plastic gloves inside the woolen ones, causing a further problem in my sensation of touch. There was also an uneven fiber pad under the soles of the shoes that caused further difficulty in my movement and an obvious distraction in my attention. Therefore, the effects produced in a cumulative way make one realize the real-life situation of a person with dementia.

At this point of discussion, I want to mention a few points on the *virtual dementia tour*. First, though the total experience is new to me, the concept is not new for me. In my childhood, we used to play "kana-machi" (Bengali word), where a child with closed eyes (with a black handkerchief wrapped around their eyes) had to find other children surrounding them. We played that challenging game with joy but could not realize the real-life significance of it in those days. Although the vision was blocked, other senses were very sharp at that age. For me, the experience of the *virtual dementia tour* at this age was a realization of the concept of an old memory. Second, as I have mentioned earlier, the time span of the *virtual dementia tour* should be a few minutes longer so that the participants can experience it better. Finally, I have confusion regarding one piece of equipment used here. In India, "acupressure" is used as a therapeutic intervention. In that therapy, pressure is applied to some particular areas, mainly on the sole (and palm), which stimulates specific sensory nerve endings, and thereby through some endocrine secretion and blood flow regulation, it relieves the symptoms. Therefore, sensory stimulation is used as a positive approach here. Nevertheless, in the *virtual dementia tour*, the ridges on the fiber pad exert pressure on some particular areas on the sole to create a negative effect so that the participants can feel a sensation that resembles the feelings of a person with dementia. I am still confused by whether there are some overlapping areas in these two concepts. In my opinion, the *virtual dementia tour* is an outstanding innovation by P. K. Beville. This knowledge is a step ahead in the present world of dementia, and as a social worker, I am very happy and excited about this experience. However, at the same time, as a medical professional, I expected more from the program.

7.6 Management of Dementia: Common Practices and Their Challenges

Persons with chronic health problems like dementia need regular care and support from other people. This support usually comes from two broad sources, either from coresident family members or from various formal caregivers of different professions. According to a recent study, the current number of dementia patients is likely to increase by 300% in the next four decades (Ferri et al., 2005). On the other hand, currently, in the US healthcare system, there is a massive shortage of trained workforce in dementia caregiving (Institute of Medicine, 2015). This situation is more or less the same across the globe. So, there is confusion that always exists regarding the management of a dementia patient. It is not only the general population that suffers from this deficiency of awareness regarding the conception of dementia, but healthcare providers also do not handle many cases in their practice because there is no significant emphasis on the diagnosis and management of dementia in the training of healthcare providers. Moreover, irrespective of various government and nongovernmental organizations, institutional management may apply a "one-size-fits-all" approach to improving dementia care, while dismissing the notion that individuals differ in treatment needs. Most of these persons often represent complete anosognosia. Many clinicians cannot rectify that; by focusing on the deficits, they may unintentionally and wrongfully communicate that the person has declined and is of no value in society. In general, people assume signs of dementia to be the same as aging. This notion largely affects the management of a person with dementia. Due to their cognitive impairment, persons with dementia usually are not able to provide for their day-to-day necessities, which puts them at increased risk for wandering, falls, infection, malnutrition, and being exploited by others. For these persons, dementia also makes it harder to detect abuse.

Often, we encounter persons with dementia, either in our own family or in our close neighbor circle or intimate friend circle. Most of the time, the other family members (having persons with dementia) wonder what they should do. We all have a busy life schedule; we do not find any opportunity to provide full-time care for these helpless individuals. Often, we hesitate to decide whether it is better to move a senior with dementia to an assisted living facility (or old-age homes) for better management by professional caregivers or to keep the person in his/her own comfortable place with the risk of getting improper and unprofessional care. Identifying these unique challenges expressed by the growing number of residents with dementia, many institutional settings (especially the assisted living facilities) now offer special care units for persons with dementia (Zimmerman & Sloane, 2007).

However, in any environment, persons with dementia should be protected from exploitation, like neglect, abuse, and harm, which may occur knowingly (due to revengeful or casual approach from the caregiver) or unknowingly (accidentally). Environments should be safe, clean, and free of hazards that may not be known or recognized by persons with dementia. There should be secured perimeters with locked doors and gates in institutional settings, restricted resident access to sharp and toxic objects, additional fire alarms in dementia care units, and enough supports (like handrails) in walking places like corridors and stairs (even in bathrooms). Staff should be sufficient in number, including physicians and nurses, and adequately trained with dementia-specific programs and services to provide well-being for individuals with dementia. There must be strict medication management; under no circumstances should a resident be sedated or chemically restrained. The states should establish a basic standard regarding environmental safety, staffing, and chemical restraint use and periodically revisit these regulations and strategies to ensure the implementation of those policies (Kaskie et al., 2015).

Elder abuse is another challenge in providing an optimal level of care for older adults. Persons with dementia commonly experience health abuse or harm. Person-centered care requires the active involvement of the persons with dementia themselves. When the capacity of an individual to direct their own daily routine changes due to dementia or other chronic conditions, they become victimized more easily. This abuse may come in the form of over- or underdose of conventional medication, excessive use of sedatives, and sexual or emotional harassment. These cause worsening of the person's physical or mental condition, producing faulty medical bills, or even neglecting daily activities that require assistance and may affect nutrition, hygiene, or even rest. The caregivers should realize the feelings of those persons and should be concerned about their attitude toward those persons. Abuse appears to occur most often in domestic home situations and may be perpetrated by adult caregivers, family caregivers, or other persons (Bond & Butler, 2013). It may also occur in institutional settings such as long-term care facilities, nursing homes, or hospices (Jayawardena & Liao, 2006). Elder abuse is now considered a silent epidemic; one in every nine Americans over 60 years of age has experienced abuse. Only 1 in 23 cases are reported. The experience of elder abuse is showing an increasing trend among persons with dementia (Dong et al., 2014).

Dementia is an outcome of different diseases, such as Alzheimer's disease, Parkinson's disease, and post-cerebrovascular accidents. However, most of the diseases causing dementia are progressive, which means that the persons with the disease only get worse over time. As there is no specific curative management available for dementia, the drugs only used for symptomatic relief can slow the progression of disease. Most of these costly drugs have some efficacy but limited effectiveness for most patients (Casey et al., 2010). Common adverse effects of these medicines are feeling sick, muscle cramps, tiredness, syncope, headache, diarrhea (anticholinesterase inhibitors like donepezil and rivastigmine), dizziness, drowsiness, breathing difficulty, and high blood pressure (memantine). Therefore, these should be used with extreme caution and with frequent monitoring of different blood parameters. The treatment is to be continued as long as it is thought to be worthwhile and must be reviewed periodically by a specialist care team. Often these patients are likely to be on numerous medications due to the concurrent existence of multiple comorbid conditions. This is the responsibility of both informal caregivers and healthcare providers to ensure that patients are taking those medicines properly (Poland et al., 2014). Maintaining an updated record of medication is essential for these individuals. This involves keeping a list of medicines in an easily accessible location and whether the person is taking dietary/herbal products, which may cause drug interference. The measures also involve whether the person is having any problem taking the medication, which may lead to over- or underdosing and may cause undesirable side effects. But, practically, maintaining all of these together is impossible in most cases, so they are only of limited value.

Therefore, dementia has no definite curative intervention through modern medications available to date. In this context, a person-centered approach to care shifts the mindset of care partners from a traditional medical model to a promising social model in the management of dementia, where personal autonomy, choice, comfort and dignity, and purposeful living are maintained (Desai et al., 2017). As the number of persons with dementia receiving institutional care increases gradually, the significance of person-centered care also increases day by day. The progression of the disease process in dementia varies depending on the underlying disease; even this varies by person and their ability to cope with different comorbidities. In some, the onset of cognitive decline may be slow, while this decline shows rapid progression in others. Similarly, the behavioral, psychological symptoms and the family and social environments also differ from person to person (Molony et al., 2018). Several discrete factors determine the actual mental state of a person with dementia, and those can be discerned only through detailed observation (Fazio et al., 2018). Therefore, the evaluation of every person with dementia is different, and management should be individualized according to the person's needs and living environment to provide optimal care (Takeda et al., 2012). Some scholars consider that in managing dementia, the medical model emphasizes deficits and loss; however, person-centered care focuses on individual experience and remaining strengths and abilities and potential positive interactions with others (Fazio et al., 2018; Power, 2010). Loneliness, helplessness, and boredom are three major elements responsible for most of the sufferings of older adults (Desai & Grossberg, 2001; Thomas, 1996). Dr. Bill Thomas first introduced the term "the three plagues" to indicate loneliness, boredom, and helplessness. Loneliness is the unpleasant sensation felt when an individual wants companionship but cannot get it (Thomas, 1996). Mother Teresa described this scary feeling among most older adults as the most terrible poverty: "Loneliness and the feeling of being unwanted is the most terrible poverty" (Berg-Weger & Morley, 2020, p.244). Loneliness generates from the scanty social contact and from the absence of persons available to share social and emotional experiences. It is a common feeling of older adult residents in different long-term care facilities and occurs as a consequence of various personal losses experienced by them. These losses may be of the companionship of family and friends or autonomy and self-identity. Loneliness has a significant impact on both the physical and mental well-being of older adults, especially in long-term care settings; it is associated with increased blood pressure, sleep disturbances, depression, and anxiety (Cacioppo & Hawkley, 2009). According to Thomas (1996), helplessness is the sensation of pain felt by an individual when (s)he receives persistent care and support; however, the individual has a minimal opportunity to contribute to others, whereas boredom is the pain felt when individuals' life becomes monotonous and lacks spontaneity. If residents feel bored during any phase of management, the concerned caregivers experience burnout. Therefore, we need to promote joyous feelings in these people (Fazio et al., 2018). Respecting the wisdom and experiences of older adults, we need to support them to find ways to contribute to their communities and social groups based on strengths, past experiences, and social engagement.

Different psychosocial practices are showing encouraging results in reducing behavioral and psychological symptoms of dementia (BPSD) and improvement in the quality of life for persons with dementia (Fazio et al., 2018). Common behavioral and psychological strategies include engaging the persons with dementia with validation therapy, reminiscence therapy, music therapy, pet therapy, engagement through loving companionship, and other meaningful activities (Scales et al., 2018). Cognitive training is the technique to improve one's neurological decline used for rehabilitation purposes in various cognitive problems, including stroke and Alzheimer's disease. Neuroplasticity is the main factor considered behind cognitive training. Current "alternative joy practice," promoted by the Eden Alternative model, suggests engaging older adults in various meaningful and spontaneous activities. In this regard, cognitive rehabilitation therapy is a behavioral model to manage persons with cognitive impairment to improve cognitive skills through the continuous practice of compensatory activities (Choi & Twamley, 2013). Engagement as a part of cognitive rehabilitation therapy is also considered a tool used to mitigate worsening cognitive incapability (Choi & Twamley, 2013). It was a wonderful experience to watch a validation therapy by the renowned therapist Naomi Feil (memorybridge, 2009) with her client who has dementia. In this person-centered interaction, Feil, regardless of her religious affiliation as Jewish, was able to connect with her client, 87-year-old Gladys Wilson, on a spiritual level. Feil sang "Jesus Loves Me" in front of Gladys repeatedly until Gladys responded to her and sang along with the same rhythm. As part of her therapy, Feil also used touch, a nontraditional practice in psychotherapeutic interventions. However, by singing along and touching her in a nurturing way, Feil became a symbol for Gladys's mother and helped her feel validated as a fellow human being.

7.7   Complementary and Alternative Approaches: A Promising Option

The significance of an alternative approach to dementia is emerging as a great option. "The usefulness and safety of complementary and integrative health interventions and their roles in improving health and healthcare" are already established (National

Center for Complementary and Integrative Health, 2016). Complementary and alternative medicine (CAM) has a potentially significant role in the management of dementia, and the use of these strategies in the United States is increasing rapidly (Lavretsky, 2009). According to the American Cancer Society, complementary and alternative medicine is defined as "supportive methods used to complement evidence-based treatment. Complementary therapies do not replace mainstream treatment and are not promoted to cure disease. Rather, they alleviate symptoms and improve well-being and quality of life" (Takeda et al., 2012). It can be assumed that the perceived helpfulness of complementary and alternative approaches is similar to that of conventional therapies (Lavretsky, 2009). A national US survey noted a 47% increase in total visits to complementary and alternative medicine practitioners, from 427 million in 1990 to 629 million in 1997 (Lavretsky, 2009). In some places, these so-called nontraditional approaches are used with existing conventional medical management (complementary), and in other places, they are used alone (alternative). The beneficial role of complementary and alternative health interventions and their effectiveness on the outcomes of health status and aging well are already established (National Center for Complementary and Integrative Health, 2016). Currently, different complementary and alternative practices are used, such as using natural products, Ayurveda (ancient Indian herbal medication), yoga and meditation (mindfulness practices), chiropractic manipulation, dietary modification with different food items, laughter therapy, and music therapy (Desai & Grossberg, 2001; National Center for Complementary and Integrative Health, 2016). It has been studied that performing intellectually demanding activities is more beneficial to have a cognitive-stimulating function (Stine-Morrow et al., 2014); on the other hand, activities that require the least cognitive stimulation may lead to future cognitive decline (Wang et al., 2006).

Meaningful engagement in everyday life is essential for individual well-being, and it enhances the quality of life for persons with dementia (Cohen, 2006). Mindful practice in several areas has promising roles in supporting the quality of life for people living with dementia. Yoga is an ancient Indian technique of interactive mind-body practice, which is a combination of physical activity (posture) with mindfulness practices (breath control) and meditation. Yoga has a down regulatory effect on the sympathetic nervous system and the hypothalamus-pituitary-adrenal axis in response to stress (Hariprasad et al., 2013; Ross & Thomas, 2010). This effect has a substantial impact on the major neurotransmitters, such as dopamine and serotonin. This also reduces neuroinflammation and improves cognition (Ross & Thomas, 2010), thereby potentially preventing dementia. Depression is considered a potentially modifiable risk factor for dementia. Yoga has been proven to have a cognitive-enhancing property and inhibits depression (Mathersul & Rosenbaum, 2016). Chronic stress and depression, along with cognitive impairments, form a vicious cycle that further deteriorates the condition of persons with dementia. Yoga and meditation have a huge importance in this context. By reducing inflammation, blood pressure, heart rate, and respiration rate and affecting the hypothalamus-pituitary-adrenal axis, meditation has a promising role as a cost-effective and safe intervention in older adults with cognitive impairment (Innes & Selfe, 2014). More than that, it is not only beneficial for dementia; instead, it also helps in various other physical and mental disorders, mostly generated due to oxidative stress. Furthermore, research also suggested that the effect sizes reflecting the effect of yoga intervention on various cognitive domains ranged from 0.30 to 0.39, even in participants with mild cognitive impairment and dementia (Bhattacharyya et al., 2021). These effect sizes are very close to those observed in various randomized controlled trials aiming to measure the efficacy of cholinesterase inhibitors such as donepezil (Knight et al., 2018; Rockwood, 2004) in participants with a similar level of cognitive impairment. The research, showing this effect, combined with having no adverse effects and a wide range of benefits beyond cognition, underscores the potential utility of yoga intervention in maintaining cognition.

Though the way "yoga" is practiced now, in my opinion, is just a mere "modification of yoga" for the twenty-first century, we are using it only for commercialization, more to popularize ourselves than to popularize *yoga*. We are using *yoga* just as a "package," consisting of some physical exercises along with a few breathing practices. However, *yoga* is much more than that; it has much more potency, not only in relieving many diseased conditions but also in attaining a healthy and peaceful life at any age. The practice of yoga is not that easy; to achieve a considerable outcome, we have to walk a long distance. Three obvious questions should come to our mind before we proceed with every step; those are "who," "how," and "why"? Answers to the first couple of questions are straightforward; however, the last question is one that's probably unanswered for most of us, even to date. We are blindly doing many things floating with the trends, but we should know the answer to "why" before depending on yoga. As the first step, we must learn the philosophy behind *yoga* from ancient Indian literature.

7.8 Conclusion

Management of dementia is a social problem that requires socially meaningful solutions, which include a tailored, individualized approach to care involving minimal antipsychotic medication (Coffey, 2019). I always believe that until and unless extreme necessity arises, persons with dementia should be cared for within their known and comfortable home atmosphere. Support and consultation may be needed from one or more healthcare or paramedical professionals, depending on the severity and individual needs of the concerned person with dementia. It should be assured that the person with dementia gets proper and balanced nutrition and adequate hydration. Dopaminergic food items, such as turmeric, almonds, dark chocolate, blueberries, and bananas, must be incorporated into the daily dietary items. In addition, persons with dementia must be engaged in some physical activities, like yoga (physical exercises and breathing exercises), and they must have social connections. Family member's company and participation are proven to have the most significant help to overcome the barrier of dementia. This awareness generation within society is also the responsibility of every healthcare provider.

References

Alzheimer's & Related Disorders Society of India. (2010). *The dementia India report: prevalence, impact, costs and services for dementia: Executive summary* (Shaji, K. S., Jotheeswaran, A. T., Girish, N., Bharath, S., Dias, A., Pattabiraman, M, & Varghese, M, Eds.). ARDSI, New Delhi. ISBN.

Alzheimer's Association. (2017). Alzheimer's disease facts and figures. *Alzheimers & Dementia, 13*, 325–373. https://doi.org/10.1016/j.jalz.2017.02.001

Alzheimer's disease International. (2015). *World Alzheimer's report: The global impact on Dementia. An analysis of prevalence, incidence, cost, and trends.* Retrieved from: https://www.alz.co.uk/research/WorldAlzheimerReport2015.pdf

Barry, L. C., & Byers, A. L. (2016). Risk factors and prevention strategies for late-life mood and anxiety disorders. In K. W. Schaie & S. L. Willis (Eds.), *Handbook of psychology of aging* (8th ed., pp. 409–427). Academic.

Bhattacharyya, K. K., Andel, R., & Small, B. J. (2021). Effects of yoga-related mind-body therapies on cognitive function in older adults: A systematic review with meta-analysis. *Archives of Gerontology and Geriatrics, 93*, 104319. https://doi.org/10.1016/j.archger.2020.104319

Berg-Weger, M., & Morley, J. (2020). Loneliness in old age: An unaddressed health problem. *The Journal of Nutrition, Health & Aging, 24*(3), 243–245. https://doi.org/10.1007/s12603-020-1323-6

Beville, P. K. (2017, September 18). *Virtual dementia tour. Event conducted at Gerontology Institute.* Georgia State University.

Bond, M. C., & Butler, K. H. (2013). Elder abuse and neglect: Definitions, epidemiology, and approaches to emergency department screening. *Clinics in Geriatric Medicine, 29*(1), 257–273. https://doi.org/10.1016/j.cger.2012.09.004

Brewster, P. W. H., Melrose, R. J., Marquine, M. J., Johnson, J. K., Napoles, A., MacKayBrandt, A., Farias, S., Reed, B., & Mungas, D. (2014). Life experience and demographic influences on cognitive function in older adults. *Neuropsychology, 28*(6), 846–858.

Cacioppo, J. T., & Hawkley, L. C. (2009). Perceived social isolation and cognition. *Trends in Cognitive Sciences, 13*, 447–454.

Casey, D. A., Antimisiaris, D., & O'Brien, J. (2010). Drugs for Alzheimer's disease: Are they effective? *Pharmacy and Therapeutics, 35*(4), 208–211.

Choi, J., & Twamley, E. W. (2013). Cognitive rehabilitation therapies for Alzheimer's disease: A review of methods to improve treatment engagement and self-efficacy. *Neuropsychology Review, 23*(1), 48–62. https://doi.org/10.1007/s11065-013-9227-4

Coffey, W. O. (2019). Dementia and Drugs: It's up to us to change the conversation. *CSA Journal, 74*(2), 12–17.

Cohen, G. D. (2006). Research on creativity and aging: The positive impact of the arts on health and illness. *The American Society on Aging, 30*, 7–15.

Desai, A. K., & Grossberg, G. T. (2001). Recognition and Management of Behavioral Disturbances in Dementia. *Primary Care Companion to the Journal of Clinical Psychiatry, 3*(3), 93–109. https://doi.org/10.4088/pcc.v03n0301

Desai, A., Wharton, T., Struble, L., & Blazek, M. (2017). Person-centered primary care strategies for assessment of and intervention for aggressive behaviors in dementia. *Journal of Gerontological Nursing, 43*(2), 9–17. https://doi.org/10.3928/00989134-20170111-07

Dong, X., Chen, R., & Simon, M. A. (2014). Elder abuse and dementia: A review of the research and health policy. *Health Affairs (Project Hope), 33*(4), 642–649. https://doi.org/10.1377/hlthaff.2013.1261

Fazio, S., Pace, D., Flinner, J., & Kallmyer, B. (2018). The fundamentals of person-centered care for individuals with dementia. *The Gerontologist, 58*(suppl_1), S10–S19. https://doi.org/10.1093/geront/gnx122

Ferri, C. P., Prince, M., Brayne, C., Brodaty, H., Fratiglioni, L., Ganguli, M., Hall, K., Hasegawa, K., Hendrie, H., Huang, Y., Jorm, A., Mathers, C., Menezes, P. R., Rimmer, E., Scazufca, M., &

Alzheimer's Disease International. (2005). Global prevalence of dementia: A Delphi consensus study. *Lancet (London, England), 366*(9503), 2112–2117.

Gawande, A. (2014). *Being mortal. Medicine and what Matters most in the end*. Metropolitan Press (ISBN: 978-1410478122).

Hariprasad, V. R., Koparde, V., Sivakumar, P. T., Varambally, S., Thirthalli, J., Varghese, M., Basavaraddi, I. V., & Gangadhar, B. N. (2013). Randomized clinical trial of yoga-based intervention in residents from elderly homes: Effects on cognitive function. *Indian Journal of Psychiatry, 55*(Suppl 3), S357–S363. https://doi.org/10.4103/0019-5545.116308

Hoyer, W. J., & Verhaeghen, P. (2006). Memory Aging. In J. E. Birren & K. W. Schaie (Eds.), *Handbook of the psychology of aging* (6th ed., pp. 209–224). Academic.

Innes, K. E., & Selfe, T. K. (2014). Meditation as a therapeutic intervention for adults at risk for Alzheimer's disease – potential benefits and underlying mechanisms. *Frontiers in Psychiatry, 5*(40). https://doi.org/10.3389/fpsyt.2014.00040

Institute of Medicine. (2015). *Retooling for an aging America: Building the health care workforce*. The National Academies Press. Available at: http://www.nap.edu. Accessed 6 Nov 2015.

Jayawardena, K. M., & Liao, S. (2006). Elder abuse at end of life. *Journal of Palliative Medicine, 9*(1), 127–136. https://doi.org/10.1089/jpm.2006.9.127

Knight, R., Khondoker, M., Magill, N., Stewart, R., & Landau, S. (2018). A systematic review and meta-analysis of the effectiveness of acetylcholinesterase inhibitors and memantine in treating the cognitive symptoms of dementia. *Dementia and Geriatric Cognitive Disorders, 45*(3–4), 131–151. https://doi.org/10.1159/000486546

Knopman, D. S., & Petersen, R. C. (2014). Mild cognitive impairment and mild dementia: a clinical perspective. *Mayo Clinic Proceedings, 89*(10), 1452–1459. https://doi.org/10.1016/j.mayocp.2014.06.019

Lavretsky, H. (2009). Complementary and alternative medicine use for treatment and prevention of late-life mood and cognitive disorders. *Aging Health, 5*(1), 61–78. https://doi.org/10.2217/1745509X.5.1.61

Lin, S., & Lewis, F. M. (2015). Dementia friendly, dementia capable, and dementia positive: Concepts to prepare for the future. *The Gerontologist, 55*(2), 237–244.

Lustig, C., & Lin, Z. (2016). Memory: Behavior and neural basis. In K. W. Schaie & S. L. Willis (Eds.), *Handbook of the psychology of aging* (8th ed., pp. 147–163). Academic Press.

Kaskie, B., Nattinger, M., & Potter, A. (2015). Policies to protect persons with dementia in assisted living: Déjà Vu all over again? *The Gerontologist, 55*(2), 199–209. https://doi.org/10.1093/geront/gnu179

Mantri, S., Fullard, M., Gray, S. L., Weintraub, D., Hubbard, R. A., Hennessy, S., & Willis, A. W. (2019). Patterns of dementia treatment and frank prescribing errors in older adults with Parkinson disease. *JAMA neurology, 76*(1), 41–49. https://doi.org/10.1001/jamaneurol.2018.2820

Mathersul, D. C., & Rosenbaum, S. (2016). The roles of exercise and yoga in ameliorating depression as a risk factor for cognitive decline. *Evidence-Based Complementary and Alternative Medicine, 2016*, 4612953. https://doi.org/10.1155/2016/4612953

Memorybridge. (2009, May 26). *Gladys Wilson and Naomi Feil*. [Video]. YouTube. https://youtu.be/CrZXz10FcVM

Molony, S. L., Kolanowski, A., Van Haitsma, K., & Rooney, K. E. (2018). Person-centered assessment and care planning. *The Gerontologist, 58*(suppl_1), S32–S47. https://doi.org/10.1093/geront/gnx173

National Center for Complementary and Integrative Health. (2016). *Complimentary, alternative or integrative health: What's in a name?* U.S. Department of Health and Human Services. Retrieved from: https://nccih.nih.gov/health/integrative-health#cvsa

Poland, F., Mapes, S., Pinnock, H., Katona, C., Sorensen, S., Fox, C., & Maidment, I. D. (2014). Perspectives of carers on medication management in dementia: lessons from collaboratively developing a research proposal. *BMC Research Notes, 7*, 463. https://doi.org/10.1186/1756-0500-7-463

Power, G. A. (2010). *Dementia beyond drugs: Changing the culture of care*. Health Professional Press (ISBN 978-1-932529-56-2).

Rockwood K. (2004). Size of the treatment effect on cognition of cholinesterase inhibition in Alzheimer's disease. *Journal of Neurology, Neurosurgery, and Psychiatry, 75*(5), 677–685. https://doi.org/10.1136/jnnp.2003.029074

Ross, A., & Thomas, S. (2010). The health benefits of yoga and exercise: A review of comparison studies. *Journal of Alternative and Complementary Medicine, 16*(1), 3–12.

Saxon, S., Etten, M., & Perkins, E. (2015). *Physical change & aging; A guide for the helping profession* (6th ed.). Springer.

Scales, K., Zimmerman, S., & Miller, S. J. (2018). Evidence-based nonpharmacological practices to address behavioral and psychological symptoms of dementia. *The Gerontologist, 58*(suppl_1), S88–S102. https://doi.org/10.1093/geront/gnx167

Stine-Morrow, E. A., Payne, B. R., Roberts, B. W., Kramer, A. F., Morrow, D. G., Payne, L., Hill, P. L., Jackson, J. J., Gao, X., Noh, S. R., Janke, M. C., & Parisi, J. M. (2014). Training versus engagement as paths to cognitive enrichment with aging. *Psychology and Aging, 29*, 891–906. https://doi.org/10.1037/a0014341

Takeda, M., Tanaka, T., Okochi, M., & Kazui, H. (2012). Non-pharmacological intervention for dementia patients. *Psychiatry and Clinical Neurosciences, 66*, 1–7. https://doi.org/10.1111/j.1440-1819.2011.02304.x

Taylor, C. A., Greenlund, S. F., McGuire, L. C., Lu, H., & Croft, J. B. (2017). Deaths from Alzheimer's Disease — United States, 1999–2014. *MMWR. Morbidity and Mortality Weekly Report, 66*(20), 521–526. https://doi.org/10.15585/mmwr.mm6620a1

The American Geriatrics Society. (2016). The Geriatrics Workforce Policy Studies Center (GWPS). Available at: http://www.americangeriatrics.org/advocacy_public_policy/gwps/gwps_faqs/id:3188. Accessed 25 Jan 2016.

Thomas, W. H. (1996). *Life worth living: How someone you love can still enjoy life in a nursing home: The Eden Alternative in action*. Vander Wyk & Burnham.

Wang, J. Y. J., Zhou, D. H. D., Li, J., Zhang, M., Deng, J., Tang, M., Gao, C., Li, J., Lian, Y., & Chen, M. (2006). Leisure activity and risk of cognitive impairment: The Chongqing aging study. *Neurology, 66*, 911–913. https://doi.org/10.1212/01.wnl.0000192165.99963.2a

Zimmerman, S., & Sloane, P. D. (2007). Definition and classification of assisted living. *The Gerontologist, 47*, 33–39.

Chapter 8
Aging and Diversity

8.1 Diversity and Health

For obvious reasons, as the population is becoming more diverse, some of the unique psychological, health, and social challenges represented by issues like successful aging, morbidity, and mortality are emerging gradually as matters of concern. Most of these are particularly critical for different minority populations and ultimately aid in shaping their long-term care experiences. The socioeconomic inequalities and health status in the United States are interesting to many researchers, as the country is considered the largest democracy in the present world. On the other hand, in another popular democracy, India, the socioeconomic structure and healthcare sectors have nearly similar diversity, thus attracting researchers often to make comparisons between the two countries. Health is probably the most diverse sector in any country's perspective. Also, it is not uncommon to find in every discussion topic related to diversity and aging that the common factor is health. Without having different health issues, probably any population in the world could not be diverse. Our birth is related to health, our life struggle is related to health, and our death is all about health.

One obvious question probably comes to mind, "if we are all created equally, then why am I treated differently?" (Baker, 2018). The renowned anthropologist George Murdock once defined the *family* as "The social group characterized by common residence, economic cooperation, and reproduction. It includes adults of both sexes, at least two of whom maintain a socially approved sexual relationship, and one or more children, own or adopted, of the sexually cohabiting adults" (Georgas, 2003, p.4). Globalization and urbanization have a profound influence on the transition of the traditional extended family system to the nuclear family systems of the United States. Between 2000 and 2050, in the United States, it is projected that the White older adult population will be doubled, while the older adult population of the African American community will be quadrupled. During this

© The Author(s), under exclusive license to Springer Nature Switzerland AG 2021   101
K. K. Bhattacharyya, *Rethinking the Aging Transition*,
https://doi.org/10.1007/978-3-030-88870-1_8

period, the older adult population of Asian Americans will rise to 6.5 times their current numbers (US Bureau of the Census, 2000). This growth has great importance in healthcare here. Disparities in various major disease management could be improved through social support provided by family and friends (Rooks & Thorpe, 2014). In the past four or five decades, the number of marriages among Black Americans is showing a declining pattern (Taylor et al., 2014). As spouses act as primary caregivers to their partners or other family members, in this regard, current Black older adults are facing helpless conditions. Diversity in socioeconomic status is intimately related to health inequities and health disparities (Farmer & Ferraro, 2005). With the ideology of equity, we are fighting in our everyday life for equality regarding healthy living, liberty, and the pursuit of happiness; however, the reality is entirely different. Economic stability, neighborhood and physical environment, health and healthcare, and social and community context greatly influence various health outcomes, such as mortality, morbidity, life expectancy, health status, functional limitations, and the quality of life. Therefore, policies should attain such a practical level that social and institutional inequities can be minimized and can regulate living conditions, risk behaviors, and morbidities in a more positive way.

8.2   Diversity and Its Determinants

The change in age structure is commonly referred to as a change in fertility and mortality rates. Fertility, mortality, and migration are intimately associated with the aging population. While fertility (expressed as birth rate) and mortality (death) are natural changes, migration, i.e., immigration (coming to live permanently to a different country) and emigration (leaving a country permanently), is not considered a natural phenomenon. While, on the one hand, birth and immigration add numbers to the population, death and emigration lower the size of the population, which ultimately impacts population growth/aging in the long run. Apparently, a reduction in fertility causes the population to be older, and an increase in fertility adds more children to the population; thereby, the population becomes younger. On the other hand, a decrease in old-age mortality causes the population to be older; however, reduced young-age mortality causes increased younger generations in the society. Over the long term, the scenario may change due to the influence of migration. The number and age of migrating people sometimes determine the average age of the population in the society.

In some countries, such as the United States, migration also plays an enormous role in the demographic dividend. The demographic dividend is the growth in a country's economy as a result of a change in the age structure of that country's population, especially when the share of the working-age population is greater than the nonworking-age share of the population. The United States gained a huge demographic dividend in the post-World War II period by the increasing population of the baby boomers. Unfortunately, that dividend is gradually losing importance due to the rising older adult population in this country. Currently, non-Hispanic Whites are the majority in the US population, with an average age of 42 years. Also, among the immigrants, unauthorized immigrants are mostly Hispanic, whereas legal immigrants are mostly from Asian countries. Although immigrants cause a reduction in the average age of the population (as most immigrants are of working age), this population displosion also has some mixed effects on the US economy. As most illegal immigrants are less skilled, US productivity may fall in the near future; skill shortage may impede competitiveness. Eventually, when these age groups further grow toward elderhood, population aging may become financially burdensome. Healthcare costs may increase, social welfare dependency may rise, and the demographic dividend may show a massive fall.

Also, the patterns of migration in the United States are very different. *Ethnoburb* is a common term nowadays. Most Asian (including Indian) older adults prefer to stay in a neighborhood where they can find their comfortable cultural environment, medical and social support, and ethnic similarities (Kelley-Moore & Thorpe, 2014). A unique traditional cultural heritage plays a significant role among Indians regarding the utilization of informal and formal care and championship, the influence of available social networks, proper utilization of long-term care facilities, filial piety, and coping with caregiver burden. Older adults have to face different chronic comorbidities and disabilities in later stages of life, where more dependency is required. The significance of the traditional extended family is important here. Indians consider religion as an integral part of their lives, providing a psychological resource for coping with life stressors. Asian Indian older adults report that religion imparts meaning and purpose to stressful life events like different chronic disease conditions. Extended family culture also exists in African American culture. In a study, Banks et al. (1989) delineated that Black older adults with different chronic diseases and living within the multigenerational extended family felt very lonely. They did not find enough works to be engaged and found themselves without having enough companions.

On the other hand, church-based social support has direct and mediated effects on different health and psychosocial outcomes (Krause et al., 2002). Medicare and Medicaid have a significant role in the US healthcare system. Initially, Medicare was not started to abolish racial disparities. Still, later, due to political aggression and social circumstances, it became evident in this regard also, and sudden enhancement in the number of Asian and Hispanic immigrants made this issue more complex in the context of health disparities (Weech-Maldonado et al., 2014). Although Medicare and Medicaid have gained better acceptance than what they were in the past, at least in the domain of routine and emergency management, they still are not universally accepted regarding complex and costly interventions (Weech-Maldonado et al., 2014).

Health is probably the single most crucial outcome influenced by socioeconomic inequality (Braveman & Gottlieb, 2014). There is enough evidence that the association between socioeconomic inequality and health (here, we are more concerned about older adults) is bidirectional, i.e., having a direct impact on the other. Health is also correlated with age and education status (we should consider wisdom as a factor); in general, educational attainment through greater health literacy reduces age-related morbidity and mortality. Diversities in age, sex, racial pattern, family structure, education level, and marital status influence the association between socioeconomic status and health. Cumulative inequality theory is ideal for describing these all-around health inequalities persisting due to systematic disadvantages over time (Taylor et al., 2020). Race has a significant relationship with education and employment status that impacts health outcomes. As education levels increase, Black adults do not experience the same improvement in self-rated health as White adults; furthermore, both race and socioeconomic status have been found to influence health status over time, especially in the context of the United States (Boen, 2016; Farmer & Ferraro, 2005). It is essential to focus on education through mass awareness programs because this is the only available option for our betterment in any domain in this corrupted political environment globally. However, awareness generation is not that easy. From the context of the United States, migration plays a vital role. Furthermore, this is a global problem, and we must acknowledge other colors that exist between the two extremes. Everyone should think about any social issue from a global perspective. Personally, I believe that the US population, especially the students, should be more aware of what is happening in the rest of the world. Future research may find many other essential factors impacting population health from a truly global perspective.

Religion in America is another diverse field that has deep roots in the immigrant experience. For many families, ethnic and religious identities have retained a particular affinity and interconnectedness across generations. These identities jointly foster the intergenerational transmission of a religious tradition. However, immigrant families, especially ethnic minority families, differ in the degree to which their racial or ethnic identities remain relevant down the generations and over time. In the United States, there has long been a synergistic association between religious institutions and the family that ensures the maintenance and reproduction of beliefs and values in society through the young individuals' moral and religious socialization (Dillon & Wink, 2007). However, the religious and spiritual lives of American people of different ages and the transmission of religious faith across generations have shown a great variation in recent years. From the perspective of substantial ethnic and religious diversity resulting from massive immigration to the United States in the last few decades, Putney et al. (2013) have studied the associations of ethnic and cultural heritage, religious identity or bonding, and the transference of a family's religious tradition across generations in eight multigenerational families from various racial and ethnic backgrounds. The authors found significantly less religious switching among ethnic families in their study compared to White families. When present, religious switching seems to be precipitated by religious disappointment, a crisis such as a divorce, and bad parent-child relationships. Overall, religious continuity across generations is the norm in most minor ethnic families. In all aspects, this intergenerational transmission gives rise to cultural pluralism.

In this regard, O'Rand (2016) suggested that early disadvantages are a negative risk factor across the stages of life, and the differences generated from the initial disadvantages are intensified over time. The effects of early childhood adversity are not very easy to overcome. The impact of early childhood physical and social deprivation on psychological development is profound, and also these effects impact cognition and other health statuses in early adolescence (Beckett et al., 2006). Very extreme early deprivation factors, such as severe poverty and social exclusion, play a significant role in the impact on the length of and specific psychological development in early childhood. The effects of deprivation on cognitive development persist in early adolescence, but there was significant improvement/catchup over time for the children (Beckett et al., 2006). However, this deprivation probably persists throughout life because memory at an early age remains the sharpest and environmental factors cannot fully erase those. As individuals move from younger age toward older age, their pattern of lifestyle and social roles change. However, the exact age reflected for a particular activity is debatable. Also, genetic factors may play some role here. Intensive education in the early ages of childhood has shown to have a more substantial impact on cognitive and academic development. Here we should consider the status of children who faced adverse situations at the earliest ages of their lives in highly populated countries like India. Therefore, from a global point of view, the impact of early childhood adversity apparently is much more than what it looks like.

Intraindividual variability refers to the range of small fluctuations in behavior within persons that does not occur due to systematic changes; instead, it depends on the effects of practice, learning, and developmental factors. Variability within persons may take place across tasks (dispersion) and across time (inconsistency) (Schmiedek et al., 2010). Some researchers claim that this is linked to a specific age range (Schmiedek et al., 2010). Though the influences of day-to-day variability on overall observed variability are small, still reliable and older adults show more consistent levels of everyday performance. The changes in the educational system (even the educational attainment in childhood and adolescence) and gender differences have a significant impact on the cohort differences in physical health and cognitive functions. Personality traits also play a role as a factor. Societal role changes of females, i.e., an increase of women in the workforce, accompanied by an increase in their educational levels followed by structural changes in the labor market, especially after World War I, played a significant factor in this domain. Globalization and labor policies (including health and retirement benefits) of different countries are the major factors that influence the growing inequalities among aging cohorts across countries. Also, the advances in electronic devices over time influenced cohort differences negatively regarding numerical ability. Many studies suggested that historical transitions and big societal events (many of those were culture-based) cumulatively affected individual development, ultimately shaping cohort differences related to health outcomes (Hueluer et al., 2019; Schaie et al., 2005).

The concept of generation is another important guideline in understanding cohort differences. Alwin (2013) argued that the term "generation" has at least three legitimate uses of the concept in human development research. Despite having distinct meanings, they are united by a common terminology, and various factors involving generational influences converge upon the developing individual. These three critical levels of analysis, i.e., families, cohorts, and social movements or organizations, coincide within the individual's life history. Alwin (2013) considered family as the primary unit of analysis. Generations are nested within families, and they are linked through the individual's life cycle. With this perspective, intergenerational relations are critical to the transmission of culture and human development. The author argued that the earlier generation attempts to pass along cultural heritage, while at the same time preparing its children for a life in a future world. In this regard, Elder (1974) suggested that during times when family survival is at stake, the parental generation focuses on children's immediate needs, not on "future adult roles." However, Alwin assumed that parents have considerable motivation to prepare their children for the future, as well as the present, for self-preservation of the family grouping. He strongly argued that generational succession and its impact on later generations involve some combination of preserving the past and an orientation to the future. Alwin (2013) also delineated the term "generation" in the context of birth cohorts, a group of individuals born and living at about the same time frame. Demographers refer to those born during the same calendar year as members of the same birth cohort (Alwin et al., 2006). Ryder (1965) suggested reserving the term "generation" solely for designated stages in the natural line of descent within families. However, Alwin viewed that claiming just one appropriate meaning of the term is somewhat shortsighted. The existence of cohort effects and their ability to influence social changes usually depend on the nature of processes at the individual level. According to Mannheim (1952), the idea of individuals' participation in the social and histori-cal process at a given point in time is not merely for their temporal placement in historical time; instead, it recognizes their participation in social movements of their time. According to Alwin (2013), cohorts only become the critical factor when they bind with historical events and are called "generations." As per this line of thought, the unique historical and social events happening during the youth period undoubt-edly play a vital role in shaping human lives. Therefore, the utility of the concept of "generation" for present-day research on human development can ultimately lead to a stronger understanding of the linkage between the individual and society and may emerge as a significant factor responsible for diversity (Alwin, 2013).

8.3   Socioeconomic Inequality and Healthcare Utilization

In recent years, socioeconomic inequality has emerged as one of the central focuses of health in the domain of aging research. Aging is now considered not just a segre-gated process; instead, it is a continuous process that starts from even before birth. The factors associated with health, i.e., physical, psychological, social, environmen-tal, and spiritual well-being, influence people to maintain their intraindividual vari-ability. The impact is cumulative and persists throughout their life. Globalization through export-import, media publicity, and immigration pattern is continuously changing the stabilities in any sector throughout the world. Therefore, the current social structure of the United States is not only based on the social stratification in the United States alone but is also a complex, dependent, and ongoing process linked with the entire world. No country could isolate itself socioeconomically. The inequality is bidirectional and cumulative, affecting and being affected by the individual, societal, and country levels.

In the United States, baby boomers are considered a significant demographic cohort, who were born after World War II, between 1946 and 1964. During the census in 2010, the oldest baby boomers had not even turned 65 years of age. However, since then, about 10,000 individuals daily have crossed that age threshold, and by 2030, all boomers will reach at least age 65 years. Using Schneider and Ingram's framework of the social construction of target populations (1993), Hudson and Gonyea (2012) described how the social construction and the political presence of the aging cohorts in the United States have categorized, historically, the impact of new policies in this categorization and why a definite categorization of the aging baby boomer cohort might be cumbersome. Schneider and Ingram's framework (1993) concentrates on constructing the target population to comprehend policy formation and transformation. According to the framework, target populations are socially constructed and, based on this construction, receive various actions politically. Their fourfold typology illustrates how the target populations are constructed and the amount of power these populations possess. The target population in the United States was labeled as "dependents" in the pre-World War II years. At that time, older adults were considered unimportant in US societies due to their small number, poverty, and low life expectancy. Shearson (1938) first studied the economic status of older adults and found that the majority of them depended on others, at least for economic support. It was considered that their status could be corrected, and as a result, they became the targeted population for Old Age Assistance in Roosevelt's New Deal program. However, older adults' economic status in the post-World War II years changed dramatically. The older population's poverty rate continued to decline, mainly due to Social Security benefits and increased life expectancy. The "dependent" status of older adults was dramatically changed into an "advantaged" category (Hudson & Gonyea, 2012). In this period, which was described by Treas and Bengtson (1982) as "democratization of aging," many policies were enacted to benefit the elderly, including disability insurance, Medicare, the Older Americans Act, the Age Discrimination in Employment Act, and the Employee Retirement Income Security Act. During this time, political activities, including voting participation of older adults, increased remarkably. The creation of new policies and new organizations, such as the AARP (American Association of Retired Persons) and the Leadership Council of Aging Organizations, resulted from greater political involvement of older adults. On the one hand, this handed more power to them and put them into the "advantaged" category on the other (Hudson & Gonyea, 2012). Since then, the baby boomer generation is considered in the category of "contenders." While many believe in programs to assist this cohort, some do not believe the cohort still needs assistance. However, both views are concerned about the country's potential economic strains if the current level of support for the older adults continues. Studies widely documented how the baby boomer cohort's enormous size slows economic growth and increases debt and concern over resources (Hudson & Gonyea, 2012). Furthermore, many baby boomers face the challenge of not having enough income or deposit to meet their retirement needs and uninsured medical expenses. These political pressures, competition, and constraints have a compounded effect on the aging cohort to move forward as contenders, and vulnerable boomers may be downgraded back to the dependent status, seeking programs targeted to assist them. This social stratification may have a counter-effect on the various advantages that current US society possesses.

On the other hand, in India, a substantial proportion of older adults are in critical need of better support for aging well, but the available resources are not enough. Even the term *gerontology* is not very common there. After close dealings with the older adult population in India for several years, it is not very hard to realize that physical treatment alone is not enough to enhance their quality of life. The older adult dependents need a holistic management with physical and mental therapy; nutritional, behavioral, and socioeconomic support; and an easily acceptable management that enhances their quality of life.

While exploring the usage pattern of healthcare resources in the United States, the most exciting thing that I have found is the approach toward health and aging well, though this is not "new" for me. Health, to me, is always a concept of a dual character, "good health" and "bad health." In the United States, health is always considered well-being. According to the World Health Organization (1946), "Health is a state of complete physical, mental, and social wellbeing not merely the absence of disease or infirmity." I am from a country where knowledge of medicine is probably the most ancient, and ancient medicine, the "Ayurveda," is considered the mother of every treatment in the world. In today's India, the ill person is still considered a "patient." However, in the United States, the sufferer is described as a "person having a disorder." I do not know how much this impacts the disease progression, but certainly this affects the dignity of the concerned person. In the domain of medical sciences, where conventional treatment cannot offer much help for dementia, for example, a change from the traditional medical model to the experimental social model is gaining championship. The changing perception is not "new" for me, but the approach is "new." In India, we are rushing toward scientific progression, from the ancient model to technological advancement in every case, without realizing the outcome. In the United States, everything is going pragmatically. This pragmatic perception is "new" for me. These are unique concepts; future researchers should apply this knowledge. Person-centered care with the idea of "culture change" is not "new" for me, but I am surprised to see that the concept we have forgotten is being used to its fullest by perhaps the most developed country in the present world. Affirmative action in the United States is not "new" for me; in India, there is also a reservation (commonly termed as *quota*) system that still exists (even after more than 70 years of independence) based on the social caste stratification. This demarcation, once influenced by the ancient concept of the "Varnashram" system, still persists in Indian society. The minority population often dealt with various strategies in different countries, not for the benefit of minority populations only but for the benefit of the politicians, too. This idea is not "new" for me. The approaches for diverse populations in different countries are "new" for me. Keeping these concepts in mind, we need to proceed with applying them in an alternative therapeutic intervention strategy.

Although many approaches are unique in the United States, they still have some loopholes. The awareness services in the United States are too technology-dependent. If we increase the workforce and they can provide in-person care, it will be much better for the older adults, as touch always plays a bigger role than tele-interaction in building intimacy and trustworthiness. Moreover, health (particularly bad health) is very much related to the doctor-patient relationship. It is now an era of specialization. However, in our childhood, we saw so many family physicians who were not only a doctor but also were like a family member of the persons concerned. Therefore, whether it is a medical model or a social model, we should involve more physicians in every program to increase its trustworthiness among the general population. India, one of the most populous democracies in the world, possesses a unique phenomenon of "unity in diversity" due to its multilingual, multireligious, multicultural, and varied geographical background. The United States also has almost a similar environment. However, the family structure is different here. The first introduction of an individual to society begins with their family. The traditional Indian multigenerational extended family concept is not available here; in the United States, the nuclear family is the norm, and life is very self-centered. This atmosphere creates a great difference in my thought process, and this is "new" for me. Family and society have a great role in the life course of every individual, and obviously that plays a direct role in health status. Health is a "condition," not just "well-being" (I differ from the WHO concept); it is not a wish, it is a status. If the determinants are not optimal, an individual cannot always experience good health (well-being). The civilization in the United States is relatively young, and like our life course, it is currently going through its best physical and mental condition. Therefore, everything in this country is much hyped to the rest of the world; technological advancement and US dollar valuation further enhance the situation. A casual and conceited feeling of greatness among the general population always persists in the United States. They are not even bothered about natural resources and are wasting freely. Many times, this attitude is alarming. That is why immigrants are coming in waves, but soon after arriving, they realize the practical life and the struggle to survive here. This transition is enormous. For many, the transition is not only in discovering the direction of the off/on button on the electric switch plate, the sequence of colors in the traffic lights, or even the driving side on the road, but this transition also prevails in every step of life. The health system is not the "best" in the United States in comparison to the health systems of many other countries. As this segment is directly related to mortality, we are bound to take many steps. Private insurance plans are examples of these bindings. The healthcare sector is entirely different in the United States than that of India, both in the structural level of care providers and the healthcare costs of the care recipient. For example, the concept of a nursing home is totally different in these countries. In the United States, nursing home care and long-term care used to be considered the same. Nowadays, nursing homes are licensed and state-regulated healthcare institutions that provide long-term housing and round-the-clock care to functionally independent individuals, mainly frail older adults. In recent years, with the changing patterns of the long-term care sector, older adults have many more options to choose from for their long-term care needs, from home health providers to assisted living facilities. Whereas in India, nursing homes were once considered healthcare institutions only for the rich people. Currently, however, maybe due to the influence of globalization, the differences in the private healthcare sector are gradually decreasing across the globe. Any specific type of healthcare that earlier was a dream for the middle-class people is now a reality. On the other hand, public hospitals in the United States are closing at a much faster rate than hospitals overall. In major suburban areas, the number of public hospitals has already been reduced by 27% (134 to 98) in the last decade (1996 to 2002); therefore, good quality specialty care for uninsured and Medicaid-enrolled patients is emerging gradually as a challenge for many urban public hospitals (Higgins, 2005). Whereas in India, public hospitals, which are commonly called government hospitals, provide healthcare almost for free to its residents (legal Indian citizens and a large numbers of legal and illegal immigrants) at the point of use in any level of healthcare setting (primary, secondary, or tertiary). Therefore, as an international learner in the United States, this is "new" for me, even more so as I was a healthcare provider in both government and nongovernmental sectors in India.

8.4 Fundamental Rights and Diversity

Healthcare (at least at the primary level) is our fundamental right; it should not be restricted by resident or citizenship status in any country. Our choice must not be the headache of any government, but basic healthcare amenities must be. This imperfection is "new" for me. This is a realization from personal experience in the last few years since I entered the United States. So, it was not surprising to read that Hispanic and African Americans are much less interested than the majority White (Caucasian) Americans with the same diagnosis to undergo any kind of operative procedure (Carlisle et al., 1997). Likewise, regarding hospice use, the trends are lower among Blacks compared to Whites, except in the case of cancer (Weech-Maldonado et al., 2014). Minority people are somehow hesitant, confused to use resources here, even in the healthcare sector. African Americans, Hispanic Americans, and Asian Americans all hesitate to use surgical procedures and even preventive measures such as vaccination and cancer screening. In my opinion, this hesitation comes from an uncertainty that restricts them from trusting the healthcare system of this country (unless an emergency arises). This attitude is not just a case of the reluctance of minority people; the problem is rooted elsewhere. Healthcare is an emergency that everybody realizes; even if not, still who is responsible for that? It is the overall system. It is the education system that cannot make them aware. It is the economic complexity that keeps them suppressed. It is the social insecurity that makes them afraid to make a decision that must be taken for the sake of their own future, the future of their beloved ones. It is the country's failure, even if a single individual is living (legally) with the fear of health concerns due to affordability. Although there is at least some level of equality, disparities still persist according to access to healthcare (urban residents have more options than rural ones), previous higher income, and generosity of insurance plans. Therefore, the policymakers need to be aware that 53 years have passed since the inception of health insurance plans in the United States; now, the social structure is much more different than what it was in 1965. Therefore, policy needs to be reformed. There is still much room for improvement so that every resident (citizens and immigrants) can trust the society where they reside. In the way the minority population is aging rapidly, however, they will become the majority in the near future. In India, the blessing of the "reservation" (quota) system is now appearing as a curse on the general population. The US policymakers should be aware of that fact, too. The caste system in India is almost equivalent to the racial identity in the United States, which not only influences the health system but also every sector of life. So, we should plan accordingly to maintain uniformity. In India, to make the minority population capable enough to lead a better lifestyle and maintain uniformity with the majority group regarding sustaining quality of life, the *quota* or reservation system was introduced. After 70 years of independence, how long does the word "reservation" remain significant in a society, as shown (an example) in Fig. 8.1?

Now the question is, which group needs more benefit from the government? And for how long? Taking this example from one of the most populous democracies (India) in the world, how far is it pragmatic if a minority population claims that kind of benefit in the world's largest democracy (United States)?

There was a feeling of an emotional involvement while reading about "medicalization" (Simonds, 2017). It took me back to my early school years, when there was a book chapter on *technology for mankind*. Now, after so many years, we are still in a stifling condition, intricately bounded by technologies in every step of life. Patients do not trust their doctors, and vice versa; even we, the clinicians, do not trust ourselves. We hesitate to rely on our clinical knowledge; it is all about technology. A patient became a "client" (or customer!) for a doctor. There is no longer respect (and emotion) that exists in this noble relationship. Third parties are invading this relationship, and the whole system is becoming corrupted. Being a part of the system, nobody can change anything from the inside (like Newton's first law of motion). We

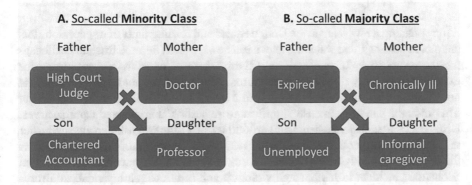

Fig. 8.1 Present reservation system in India

do not have the stamina and willpower to change anything coming out of the system. Therefore, the problem is gradually worsening. Not only hospital land but the land of every institution is also going underground with corruption and dishonesty. However, we still feel proud of our technological improvement! As a clinician, the situation was pathetic (and shameful) for me till a few months back. After coming to a so-called developed country, I realized that I was in heaven. At least there is still a chance to survive; at least the government is taking full responsibility for primary healthcare, even contributing a lot to tertiary care. But now, even asking for primary healthcare needs seems to be a luxury for us. We want to cry out for our minimum fundamental rights for existence without being certain of getting any response. Still, we are improving technologically!

We need to apply the knowledge we gained through the learning process in our future work environment. I also want to apply approaches that I learned from my traditional Indian culture to future intervention strategies for chronic conditions. Unfortunately, however, there are a few loopholes in the systems of both countries. If we can fill those gaps, it will ultimately help everyone. Although the ideal is far-fetched (maybe elusive) to implement, proceeding nearer to that aim is the most pragmatic way out. Structural barriers and cultural beliefs are significant factors influencing the health status of minority populations in this country. Awareness generation among the general population is the most important thing to do in the present circumstances to break the barrier of racial and ethnic factors. Otherwise, health will remain only medical model-oriented, as it is now. In my opinion, neither medical science nor social science alone is enough to provide the best possible aging to older adults. Therefore, if we want to maximize our efforts, we must work together. If professionals from medical science and social science work together, the idea of "aging well" will be more pragmatic. To achieve that goal, every individual needs to be a change agent; every individual should try to minimize the gap between socio-economic inequality and health, to extend a hand, along with every family, every community, and every government, for the preservation of equality, even in diversity.

8.5   Conclusion

After spending a few years in the United States and reading daily newspapers, different media postings, and watching television news, I often became frustrated to imagine the perspectives of one's country. Everywhere older adults are struggling for existence, especially if they are immigrants. Although I am not an older adult right now, I always feel anxious about my future years, when I will enter that age group. This thought has an immense significance regarding this chapter's perspectives. Different incidents are happening all around us, and often we ask ourselves whether the actions the respective authorities are taking are appropriate. Most of the time, is the country not giving enough protection to its residents? I remember one so-called "donation" incident in India; some violent youth of a local club vandalized everything in a renowned older adult couple's apartment after being refused a satisfactory monetary donation. I can clearly remember the heartrending faces of that helpless couple in the media, asking the question, "Is this our country?" So, which is our country? Where have we been born? Where are we residing now? Or where can we take a breath without any anxiety? What is the demarcation line? Language, religion, structural difference, any other human quality, or a pocketful of money? We learned in our school days that the pen is mightier than the sword. However, real life is showing us that biceps are greater than any education; politics is more powerful than any profession. Somehow every negativity seems the same as each other, everywhere, as if diversity does not exist in common people. Everywhere individuals are treated in the same way. Actual diversity exists in power, in politics, and in misusing government regulations. Power dynamics are showing changing patterns everywhere. The power of humanity becomes less and less with advancing age.

References

Alwin, D. F. (2013). Who's talking about my generation? In M. Silverstein & R. Giarrusso (Eds.), *Kinship and cohort in an aging society: From generation to generation* (pp. 133–158). Johns Hopkins University Press.

Alwin, D. F., McCammon, R. J., & Hofer, S. M. (2006). Studying baby boom cohorts within a demographic and developmental context: Conceptual and methodological issues. In S. K. Whitbourne & S. L. Willis (Eds.), *The baby boomers grow up: Contemporary perspectives on midlife*. Lawrence Erlbaum Associates.

Baker, T. A. (2018). Presidential opening and 2018 Barbara Pittard Payne lectureship in gerontology. *If we are all created equally, then why am I treated differently? Conceptualizing diversity, disparities, and health determinants collectively*. Presented at the Joint Southern Gerontological Society and the Georgia Gerontology Society Scientific Meeting, Buford, GA.

Banks, J., Cameron, W., Montague, M., Toliver, J., Hobbs, S., & Peterson, L. (1989). The chronically ill grandparent in minority multigenerational households: Problems and solutions from three points of view. *Journal of National Black Nurses' Association, 3*(2), 41–48.

Beckett, C., Maughan, B., Rutter, M., Castle, J., Colvert, E., Groothues, C., Kreppner, J., Stevens, S., O'connor, T. G., & Sonuga-Barke, E. J. (2006). Do the effects of early severe deprivation on cognition persist into early adolescence? Findings from the English and Romanian adoptees study. *Child Development, 77*(3), 696–711.

Boen, C. (2016). The role of socioeconomic factors in Black-White health inequities across the life course: Point-in-time measures, long-term exposures, and differential health returns. *Social Science & Medicine, 170*, 63–76. https://doi.org/10.1016/j.socscimed.2016.10.008

Braveman, P., & Gottlieb, L. (2014). The social determinants of health: it's time to consider the causes of the causes. *Public Health Reports (Washington, D.C.: 1974), 129*(Suppl 2), 19–31. https://doi.org/10.1177/00333549141291S206

Carlisle, D. M., Leake, B. D., & Shapiro, M. F. (1997). Racial and ethnic disparities in the use of cardiovascular procedures: Associations with type of health insurance. *American Journal of Public Health, 87*, 263–267.

Dillon, M., & Wink, P. (2007). *In the course of a lifetime: Tracing religious beliefs, practice, and change*. University of California Press.

Elder, G. H., Jr. (1974). *Children of the Great Depression*. University of Chicago Press.

Farmer, M. M., & Ferraro, K. F. (2005). Are racial disparities in health conditional on socioeconomic status? *Social Science & Medicine, 60*(1), 191–204. https://doi.org/10.1016/j.socscimed.2004.04.026

Georgas, J. (2003). Family: Variations and changes across cultures. *Online Readings in Psychology and Culture, 6*(3). https://doi.org/10.9707/2307-0919.1061

Higgins, M. (2005). *Public hospitals decline swiftly. The Washington Times.* Online Resource. Retrieved from: https://ipfs.io/ipfs/.../wiki/Public_hospital.html

Hudson, R. B., & Gonyea, J. G. (2012). Baby Boomers and the shifting political construction of old age. *The Gerontologist, 52*(2), 272–282. https://doi.org/10.1093/geront/gnr129

Hueluer, G., Ram, N., Willis, S. L., Schaie, K. W., & Gerstorf, D. (2019). Cohort differences in cognitive aging: The role of perceived work environment. *Innovation in Aging, 3*(Suppl 1), S24.

Kelley-Moore, J. A., & Thorpe, R. J. (2014). Age in place and place in age: Advancing the inquiry on neighborhoods and minority older adults. In K. E. Whitfield & T. A. Baker (Eds.), *Handbook of minority aging.* Springer.

Krause, N., Ellison, C. G., & Marcum, J. P. (2002). The effects of church-based emotional support on health: Do they vary by gender? *Sociology of Religion, 63*, 21–47.

Mannheim, K. (1952). The problem of generations. In P. Kecskemeti (Ed.), *Essays in the sociology of knowledge* (pp. 276–322). Routledge & Kegan Paul.

O'Rand, A. M. (2016). Long, Broad, and Deep: Theoretical approaches in aging and inequality. In V. L. Bengston & R. A. Settersten Jr. (Eds.), *Handbook of sociology of aging* (3rd ed., pp. 365–380). Springer.

Putney, N. M., Lam, J. Y., Nedjat-Haiem, F., Ninh, T., Oyama, P. S., & Harris, S. C. (2013). The transmission of religion across generations: How ethnicity matters. In M. Silverstein & R. Giarrusso (Eds.), *Kinship and cohort in an aging society: From generation to generation* (pp. 209–236). Johns Hopkins University Press.

Rooks, R. N., & Thorpe, R. J. (2014). Understanding age at onset and self-care management to explain racial and ethnic cardiovascular disease disparities in middle- and older-age adults. In K. E. Whitfield & T. A. Baker (Eds.), *Handbook of minority aging.* Springer.

Ryder, N. B. (1965). The cohort as a concept in the study of social change. *American Sociological Review, 30*(6), 843–861.

Schaie, K. W., Willis, S. L., & Pennak, S. (2005). An historical framework for cohort differences in intelligence. *Research in Human Development, 2*(1-2), 43–67. https://doi.org/10.1080/15427609.2005.9683344

Schmiedek, F., Lövdén, M., & Lindenberger, U. (2010). Hundred days of cognitive training Enhance Broad cognitive abilities in adulthood: Findings from the COGITO study. *Frontiers in Aging Neuroscience, 2*, 27. https://doi.org/10.3389/fnagi.2010.00027

Schneider, A., & Ingram, H. (1993). The social construction of target populations. *American Political Science Review, 87*, 334–347. https://doi.org/10.2307/2939044

Shearson, M. (1938). Economic status of the aged. *Social Security Bulletin, 1*, 5–16.

Simonds, W. (2017). *Hospital land USA: Sociological adventures in medicalization.* Routledge.

Taylor, R. J., Hernandez, E., Nicklett, E. J., Taylor, H. O., & Chatters, L. M. (2014). Informal social support networks of African American, Latino, Asian American and Native American older adults. In K. E. Whitfield & T. A. Baker (Eds.), *Handbook of Minority Aging.* Springer.

Taylor, M. G., Min, S. N., & Reid, K. M. (2020). Cumulative inequality at the end of life? Racial disparities in impairment in the time before death. *The Journals of Gerontology Series B, Psychological Sciences and Social Sciences, 75*(6), 1292–1301. https://doi.org/10.1093/geronb/gby129

Treas, J., & Bengtson, V. L. (1982). The demography of mid- and late-life transitions. *The Annals of the American Academy of Political and Social Science, 464*, 11–21. https://doi.org/10.1177/0002716282464001002

U.S. Bureau of the Census. (2000). *Projections of the total resident population by 5-year age groups, race, and Hispanic origin with special age categories: Middle series 1999–2000; middle series 2050–2070.* Retrieved from: https://www.census.gov/data/tables/2000/demo/popproj/2000-national-summary-tables.html

Weech-Maldonado, R., Pradhan, R., & Powell, M. P. (2014). Medicare and health care utilization. In K. E. Whitfield & T. A. Baker (Eds.), *Handbook of minority aging.* Springer.

World Health Organization. (1946). *Preamble to the constitution of the WHO as adopted by the International Health Conference, NY* (pp. 19–22). Author.

Chapter 9
Aging and Longevity

9.1 Impact of Longevity on the Aging Process

A twofold increase in global human life expectancy in the last century certainly indicates that the world population is "graying" (Roser, 2017). Now, we are experiencing a demographic revolution with millions of older citizens around us, and many are even centenarians (individuals of 100 years of age or older). Currently, individuals aged 85 years and older (oldest-old) are the fastest-growing cohort in the population (Cherry et al., 2013). Greater longevity is a big achievement; however, does merely adding extra years in later life influence individuals' view of aging successfully? Although this gradual and steady rise in the global older adult population could be viewed as a public health victory, supporting the notion that posits aging populations as a societal advantage and benefit, this cohort demands high-quality resources, especially regarding health and social care (Bhattacharyya et al., 2021b).

Today's world is a real challenging field for geriatricians and the healthcare system in general. Some distinct medical terminologies, like *disability*, *comorbidity*, and *frailty*, are gaining importance in recent years in the longevity research domain. *Frailty* is a physiological condition vulnerable to stress factors, characterized by weight loss, weakness, low mobility, and gait abnormality, a proportion of which increases steadily with age (Fried et al., 2004). Fried and colleagues defined *disability* as a type of physical and mental impairment limiting the essential activities of individuals required for independent living, and *comorbidity* is the coexisting condition of two or more chronic medical problems in a particular individual that increases significantly with advancing age (Fried et al., 2004). On the one hand, comorbid diseases additively may develop frailty. On the other hand, disability may well worsen frailty and comorbidity. These are specific conditions; however, each indicates different but specific care needs for older adults. The coexistence of these conditions in later life brings challenges, affecting individuals' symptoms and prognosis in a complex manner. Each condition has its significance regarding healthcare needs like hospitalization or special care assistance that affects individuals' ability to live independently. Most medical problems associated with disability, frailty, and comorbidity may be preventable, but distinct interventions are needed. As we are experiencing a sudden increase in the number of older adults in our surroundings, which was never present before, early diagnosis and proper strategies are necessary at this time for their better aging and rehabilitation in society.

With the amazing improvements in medical technologies and healthcare strategies in the last few decades, our older generations are growing toward being the old-old, oldest-old, centenarians, and even supercentenarians. In this context, the pattern of compression of morbidity in later life is very important regarding the transitioning into very old ages. It has been found that older adults, in their later ages, often delay or escape from various common age-related disorders. Evert et al. (2003) evaluated 424 centenarians and grouped them based on having 10 very common fatal disorders, such as stroke, heart diseases, non-skin malignancies, etc. The researchers categorized the centenarians based on the age of diagnosis, gender, and racial pattern and found three different morbidity profiles: survivors, delayers, and escapers. They called the first group *survivors*, those who reached their 80 years with a diagnosis of one or more chronic diseases. They used the term *delayers* to denote those who reached their 80 years without having any of those major diseases, i.e., delaying the diseases, and the term *escapers* was used to define those who attained their 100 years of age without being diagnosed with common major diseases. The researchers found that the first group had a female preponderance and the second group had a similar sex ratio, while the third group had a male preponderance. This research indicates various routes to achieve exceptional longevity. It is quite surprising that one-fifth of centenarians are reaching their current age without having major illnesses.

A study conducted in the recent past in India, where visual and hearing impairments were found to have significant effects on the lifestyles of older adults, found that people in the 80- to 100-year-old age group were predominately affected (Bhattacharyya, 2017a). Presently the growing number of older adults in India is a matter of concern in the context of humongous population explosion there; different comorbidities substantially influence the socioeconomic status of older adults in later life (Bhattacharyya, 2017a). This study was unique in its nature, as this was not carried out by any institution but instead by a family physician, who has a more intimate relationship with the families (and individuals) concerned. Thus, the data collected seems to be more authentic in nature. This community-based cross-sectional study was conducted in an urban area and surveyed 208 older adults of young-old, middle-old, and very-old age group participants. The demographic pattern revealed more males than females and more young-old than middle-old and very-old persons. Most of the participants belonged to the upper-middle class, followed by the upper-lower and lower-middle classes. Most of the older adults had multiple morbidities.

Regarding the physical health of the elderly population, visual impairment was found to be the most prevalent problem, followed by hypertension. Other than those conditions, there were also hearing impairment, musculoskeletal problems, diabetes (with complications), renal failure, and chronic obstructive pulmonary diseases that have significant influences on the lifestyle of older adults. Among psychosocial problems, depression was the most frequent problem, followed by impaired memory, intelligence, and anxiety. According to the author, the breakdown of the traditional multigenerational family into small nuclear families and the unavailability of geriatric healthcare services at the primary level of healthcare facilities are the most common causes of increasing comorbidities in the older adult population in India. The author suggested increasing awareness among older adults for regular health checkups, so that prevention and early detection of health problems can help older adults secure healthy aging and aging well. The advancement of medical technologies and treatment protocol has a profound influence on the longevity of human life, and as a result, the number of survivors is increasing day by day. However, we should also be disciplined in our lifestyles so that we can live our days of aging well as escapers because more talent is required to be an escaper. Therefore, future research is essential to relate survivors, delayers, and escapers with chronic diseases on the one hand and food habits, addiction, caregiving, mental stability, and level of resilience on the other hand. Each of these can play a vital role in the longevity of an individual, and this should be done collaboratively in varied geographical locations.

At this point in the discussion, I want to mention one of my neighbors in India, Mr. Panchanan Banerjee (name changed), who is going to be a member of the centenarian club in a month. Still, he is involved in physical activities like walking and gardening and mental activities like reading and memorizing (even banking transactions, though not online). He takes a low-calorie diet regularly but in small quantities; after taking a cold-water bath every morning, he prays in front of the deity and believes in divinity. He lives within his extended family possessing enormous power (mostly due to his vast bank savings) and gets respect from his younger family members. But most importantly, he is one of the so-called escapers who had not experienced a major disease yet. We both like each other, but he never came to my chamber, even for checking his blood pressure, because he does not believe in the allopathic system. Instead, he believes in the traditional Ayurvedic system. However, the most striking feature in his character is that he always possesses a positive outlook, and in my opinion, this is the main reason for his longevity.

9.2   Longevity from a Unique Cultural Perspective

The population of India is humongous; currently, India is the second most populous country in the world, representing a unique feature of "unity in diversity," having just over 0.6 million centenarians, with slight female preponderance (Census of India, 2011). Considering the number of centenarians, the United States, Japan, China, India, and Italy have secured their positions as the top five countries. India has a myriad of ethnicities, religions, cultures, and languages with a great amount of geographical and climatic variation. India has 22 scheduled languages (excluding multiple other local languages and more than 300 dialects across the country) used in its 29 states and 7 union territories, with a peculiar coexistence of diversity in any domain of humankind (Bhattacharyya, 2017b). From an Indian cultural perspective, longevity is considered a big public health victory; aging and wisdom are always esteemed by all. As gerontology and longevity are interrelated, the study of aging, as an interdisciplinary subject, is always considered a diverse and challenging field in research in the Indian context. Since ancient times, numerous factors are considered responsible for longevity in the Indian subcontinent; however, today's world is emphasizing more the recent medical advancements accountable for human longevity. Considering the ancient history of longevity and its spiritual connections, present-day India is still way behind in its proper recognition and representation in the rest of the world (Bhattacharyya & Molinari, 2021). In this context, this discussion is trying to find out the manifold of unique factors responsible for the longevity of Indian older adults, including centenarians.

9.2.1 Medical Advancement Versus Lifestyle Modification

In recent years, upswings in urbanization, massive signs of progress in nutrition and sanitation, breakthroughs in immunization, and availability of advanced medical amenities are considered crucial factors to have a substantial impact on human longevity globally (Finch & Tanzi, 1997). Therefore, these factors also have a profound influence on the Indian population. The discovery of newer antibiotics is showing its power over the number and pattern of infectious diseases by dramatically lowering mortality and morbidities in the older adult population. The current healthcare system in India, including the primary, secondary, and tertiary levels, is showing an upsurge in growth. Associated resources, such as health insurance, are providing an umbrella to care seekers. However, a substantial percentage of Indian older adults are still not aware of how to use the privileges of healthcare facilities (Bhattacharyya & Molinari, 2021). Accessibility to advanced healthcare facilities is still difficult for most older adults for various reasons, such as poverty, poor education, and inadequate transportation (Bhattacharyya & Molinari, 2021).

A gradual loss of social roles and recognition often denigrates older adults' social status, making them more lonely and helpless. Many feel that they themselves are practically a burden to their family members in the present socioeconomic structure. However, this is only one side of the coin. Many others want to avoid morbidity and practice different lifestyle modifications to protect themselves. Individuals try to adjust differently in their surrounding environments, where they were born and where they survive. Although many lifestyle factors both positively and negatively affect older adults' lives (Govindaraju et al., 2015), in my eyes, lifestyle modification by one's own in the way of self-discipline has a crucial role on longevity, especially from Indian older adults' perspectives.

9.2.2 Genetic Configuration Versus Positive Outlook

Research has found that human longevity is influenced by around 300–700 genes (Budovsky et al., 2013), including Apo C3-CC, FOXO3a-T, CETP-VV, and AdipoQ-del/del, which are considered to be responsible for longevity in centenarians (Barzilai et al., 2012). Govindaraju et al. (2015) suggested that genetic factors are responsible for nearly one-third of the phenotypic variations related to the trait associated with longevity, while the remaining two-thirds that are accountable for longevity consist of epigenetic and environmental determinants (Bhattacharyya & Molinari, 2021). However, in Indian culture, thoughts are rooted differently. Although many older adults suffer from several incurable diseases, they nurture their past positive episodes and their potential for the rest of their lives. This pragmatic outlook boosts them to overcome their personal losses (Amin, 2017; Dionigi et al., 2011; Lamb, 2014). Therefore, they do not always consider their aging processes as a negative consequence; instead, aging is an achievement for them, and they replenish it with dignity (Amin, 2017; Lamb, 2014).

This outlook can be described from a different context. Around 2500 BCE, one of the most ancient civilizations in human history, i.e., the Indus Valley Civilization, flourished in the northwestern part of the then Indian subcontinent (Kulke & Rothermund, 2004). This country has its own ancient culture. However, over time, a cultural conglomeration took place due to the coalescing of many other cultures, such as Muslim (Shak, Hun, Pathan, Mughal, and others) and Christian (Greek, British, Dutch, French, and others) (Bhattacharyya & Molinari, 2021). These people arrived at different periods as warriors, traders, or migrants and ultimately stayed in the country for a long time, assisting the growth of many diverse ethnic groups (Tiwari & Pandey, 2013). Consequently, many indigenous religions, such as Hinduism, Sikhism, Jainism, or Buddhism, that were born and grown here showed a great religious cohabitation with many alien religions, such as Christianity, Islam, or Persian (Bhattacharyya & Molinari, 2021). The lifestyle of Indian people reflects a peculiar endurance pattern, possibly due to this cultural acceptance from very early times. In present-day India, the majority of people are Hindu (79.8%), while Islam (14.23%), Christianity (2.30%), Sikhism (1.72%), Buddhism (0.70%), Jainism (0.36%), and others (0.9%) coexist here (Census of India, 2011). Therefore, searching for a typical genetic pattern would not yield much benefit here. Many individuals might achieve their excess longevity due to having a lucky combination of polymorphisms; however, many others may reach a similar destination with appropriate lifestyle modifications (Passarino et al., 2016). Most people who achieved an excess longevity have a positive outlook toward life; they believe in the divinity and will power to live for more years. Most of them practice self-control with a disciplined and congruous lifestyle. In my view, these have a massive impact on their longevity.

Vedas, probably the most ancient book in human civilization, portrayed individuals' desire for long life. Atharva Veda described "Pashyem sharadah shatam, Jivet sharadah shatam," which means "let me see 100 autumns, let me live 100 autumns"

(Griffith, 1899). In the Vedic era, many sages or *rishis* (spiritually wise men) worshiped God to bless them to achieve excess longevity. This is considered a cultural continuance as many older adults still prefer to bless their younger ones with similar words (Bhattacharyya, 2017b). Yogic science was so developed during that time that by maintaining a disciplined lifestyle with yoga practice, rishis could practically perceive everything in the materialistic world and even beyond that. They could perform many supernatural things, such as making themselves lighter than their actual body weight so that they can float in the air. With the stern practice of yoga and meditation, they could stop their breath, even for years, which helped them achieve excess longevity (Yogananda, 1946). Kayakalp yoga, with specific *mudra* and breathing practices, was considered to promote a longer youthful life with good health by slowing down the aging process. Those miracles were not a fluke; instead, they required immense self-control and strict practice of yoga, maybe for years. We cannot underestimate those from the mythical background only; there was enough proof and explanation in our ancient literature that all those were scientific and persisted in a real-world situation. In recent years, yoga also became popularized in the Western world. It has been proven that yoga, meditation, and other mind-body practices can prevent cognitive impairment in the long run (Bhattacharyya et al., 2021a). Alternate nostril breathing is an excellent exercise to prevent mental decline (Weiss, 1986). We must admit that yoga, along with proper lifestyle modification, had a significant impact on the well-being and life satisfaction of ancient Indian yogis.

9.2.3 Unique Features in the Indian Lifestyle for Excess Longevity

Centenarians currently exist at a more significant concentration in some specific geographic locations, i.e., blue zones. These blue zones include Okinawa in Japan, Nicoya in Costa Rica, Ikaria in Greece, Sardinia in Italy, and Loma Linda in the United States (Poulin et al., 2013). However, it has been found that centenarians lead a typical lifestyle and share a similar environment (Buettner, 2012).

9.2.3.1 Sociocultural Factors

A substantial amount of research has been conducted on centenarians in recent years. In most cases, genetic predispositions and the breakthroughs in present day's medical technologies have been emphasized as the most crucial factors for longevity, but these factors are not solely responsible for longevity among Indian centenarians (Nair, 2012). In India, cultural, familial, and spiritual beliefs (faith in a divine power is a natural phenomenon), restricted dietary habits (if a lesser amount of food is metabolized for energy, free radicals also get reduced), dietary patterns (mostly vegetarian food habits), socializing patterns (intra- and interfamily, intra- and inter-community), and regular physical and mental exercise (in daily activities) all play in a harmonious manner and help in longevity (Bhattacharyya & Molinari, 2021). Moreover, centenarians were largely self-dependent; most of them were female and widowed, coped with many setbacks in their life, and had a simple and positive outlook in mind (Ramamurti & Jamuna, 2010).

India has an opulent cultural heritage that has a strong influence on the societal infrastructure. The "Chatur-Ashram" (four stages) system originated in the Vedic era, delineating individuals' various social roles. The system is composed of "Brahmacharya," i.e., student life when one is supposed to learn, practice, and master various life education; "Grihastha," i.e., family life when one is supposed to start married life and fulfill the material needs of the conjugal life; "Vanaprastha," i.e., a transition period toward a secluded life when one is supposed to guide the next generations by educating life skills and renouncing *grihastha*; and "Sanyas," i.e., leading an ascetic life free of worldly things (Bhattacharyya & Molinari, 2021). The ashram system was established to maintain a societal discipline and a balance in individuals' life (Tiwari & Pandey, 2013). The Vedic literature depicted the stages of the ashram system as equally divided into 25 years each. Therefore, it may be assumed that individuals who experienced all stages achieved their 100-year mark and that there were many centenarians in society during that time (Bhattacharyya, 2017b). It needs to be mentioned here that the functions of individuals in the third and fourth ashrams are to deal with the supernatural power and the life within. Therefore, old age was considered ideal for intellectual activities in the Indian ashram system (Tiwari & Pandey, 2013). Two great epics of India, "The Ramayana" and "The Mahabharata," delineated several centenarian characters, along with various individual, familial, and social responsibilities of a person and the impact of the ashram system on society as a whole. Another renowned book, *Arthashastra* by Kautilya, revealed similar societal features (Bhattacharyya & Molinari, 2021).

The "caste system" was another determinant of societal life in Vedic India. It has been estimated that the caste system, which originated nearly two thousand years ago, classified individuals according to their occupational functions and unchangeable social positions, which later became a hereditary classification. The categorization comprised of "Brahmin," i.e., primarily priests and pundits; "Kshatriya," i.e., mainly warriors; "Baisya," i.e., mostly farmers and traders; and "Shudra," i.e., tenant farmers and laborers. Other than these, there was another group consisting of individuals born outside (inferior) of the caste system and grouped as "untouchable" for the other upper classes (Bhattacharyya & Molinari, 2021). Even marital arrangements are considered in the same caste, and the same tradition is continuing in today's India. The caste system was developed to maintain a stable and disciplined society many years ago, and history proves the unique and beneficial effects of the caste system on society. Since then, several changes took place in society; however, this system remained relatively unchanged due to several apparently unknown factors. Of note, today's India is suffering from many deleterious effects of the caste system that highlight its disadvantages only. Although every system needs to be modified according to contemporary perspectives, more in-depth knowledge is required for constructive criticism of the caste system.

The progression of philosophic ideas blossomed in the Vedic and post-Vedic periods. In India, the philosophical ideas are commonly termed as "Darshana," which is not precisely synonymous with its Western counterpart "philosophy" (Gupta, 2012). In the Vedic concept, *dharma* is the ideal way of life, and it does not indicate any specific population that believes a particular thought or ideology. In contrast, its literal meaning "religion" in Western countries points to some specific groups of people, such as Hindus, Muslims, Christians, and many others. As a lineage of the Vedic concept, some Hindu cultural beliefs and practices are considered integral parts of traditional "Darshanashastra." The difference between the Western idea of "religion" and the Vedic thought of "religion" often creates misconceptions regarding Indian philosophy among Western philosophers. "Of the systems of thought or darshanas, six became more famous than others, viz., Gautama's Nyaya, Kanada's Vaisesika, Kapilas Samkhya, Patanjali's Yoga, Jaimini's Purva Mimamsa and Badarayana's Uttara Mimamsa or the Vedanta" (Radhakrishnan, 1962, p. 19). All these systems were the lineages of Vedas. "The systems of thought which admit the validity of the Vedas are called astika, and those which repudiate it nastika" (Radhakrishnan, 1962, p. 20). In the contemporary era, this idea has been simplified as those individuals who believe in God are *astika* and those who do not are *nastika* (Bhattacharyya & Molinari, 2021). These concepts are commonly reflected in the thought processes of every Indian, irrespective of culture, habitat, and lifestyle.

All these factors influenced the lifestyle of Indian people, and these concepts are still significant and widespread in many communities in India. Also, from the previous discussion, it is clear that lifestyle modifications played a vital role long before the modern advancement of medications came to play its role. Simultaneously, the availability of several health systems, such as allopath, Ayurveda, yoga, siddha, homeopathy, unani, and naturopathy in India, provides a great variety to older adults for choosing their healthcare options (Bhattacharyya & Molinari, 2021). However, it has been proven that in ancient India, Ayurveda was much developed and proved to be effective on individuals' longevity.

9.2.3.2   Interpersonal Relationships

Living longer years for an individual does not always associate with living with good health, both physical and mental. Instead, in later life, older adults may face different chronic comorbidities and disabilities, which often produce increased dependency for them (Serra et al., 2011). Here comes the significance of the traditional extended family. This family culture has a significant role in longevity and aging well through emotional bonding and discipline.

Individuals experience various relationships in their life course depending on numerous social norms in India. The marital relationship is considered one of the most vital relationships in human life (Sharma et al., 2013). Accumulating evidence revealed that an excellent marital relationship causes emotional closeness that indirectly affects healthy aging and well-being in later life (Iveniuk et al., 2014; Levenson et al., 1993; Xu et al., 2015). A vast body of research suggests that compared to single individuals, married individuals tend to live longer; have reduced numbers of morbidities, such as stroke and heart attack; and face a lower risk of developing depression in later life (Shmerling, 2018; Vaillant, 2002). It has been established that some physiological and metabolic changes take place as the indirect effects of marriage are responsible for the healthy life of the concerned couple. Marriage in Indian culture is regarded as a sacred cohabitation of two individuals and a societal tie between two concerned families; this is considered an event for life (Sharma et al., 2013). "In the Hindu marriage ceremony, the bride and groom hold hands, and as a husband and wife walk seven steps (*saptapadi*) together around Agni, the Hindu God of fire, and pledge to each other their eternal friendship" (Bhattacharyya & Molinari, 2021, pp. 121–122). The fundamental concept of marriage in Hinduism is to build friendship and wish to be a trusted companion to each other in the coming days. Therefore, social norms, obeying elders, disciplined life, and fewer breakups in married life have a compound effect on individuals that helps them to achieve advantages of aging well (Fig. 9.1). Religious beliefs also come into existence here; it is believed that a good married life is the initial step of a long journey, not only in later life but also beyond that (Bhattacharyya & Molinari, 2021). This thought is considered the major cause that the divorce rate in India is around one percent, one of the lowest divorce rates compared to the rest of the world (Dholakia, 2015). This ideology in the marital relationship affects the longevity of individuals and promotes better aging (Tiwari & Pandey, 2013).

Within an Indian extended multigenerational family, most children feel comfortable with the company of their grandparents and develop a good friendship with them. The children often express their thoughts without being afraid of judgment and scolding from their grandparents. This is considered a dual relationship, where on the one hand, the grandparents play a role as an educator, friend, and companion, and on the other hand, this trustworthy and stressless relationship energizes older adults, preventing common plagues of loneliness, boredom, and helplessness. This relationship also encourages grandparents to perform various physical and mental activities that are meaningful to them and ultimately protect them from a massive risk of isolation from society. To examine the relationships between household living arrangements and the health benefits of older adults in India, Samanta et al. (2015) explored survey data of 215,754 individuals from the India Human Development Survey. They found that older adults who live within a multigenerational household possess higher health advantages compared to those in solitary living. This study proved the advantages of India's traditional multigenerational family culture that is gradually diminishing due to tremendous urbanization and consequent formation of nuclear families.

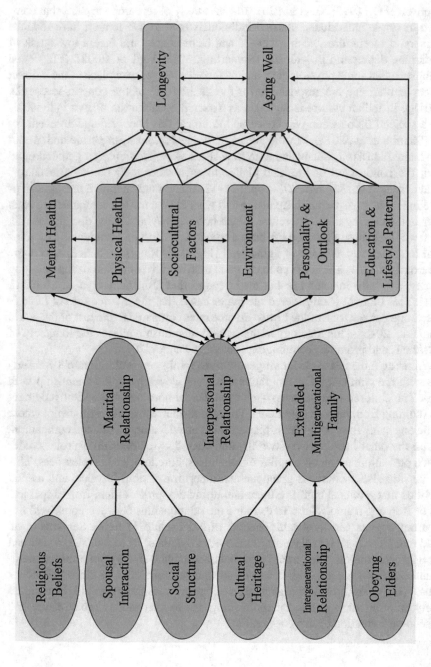

Fig. 9.1 Conceptual framework showing the association between interpersonal relationship and longevity

9.3 Conclusion

In the current socioeconomic instability, most older adults, more specifically the oldest-old individuals, struggle with the challenges of sociopolitical anxiety, malnutrition, poverty, insufficient access to healthcare, and financial uncertainty. All of these have a significant impact on the declining lifestyle of centenarians of present-day India. Globalization has a beneficial impact on the lifestyle of individuals, including older adults. Anything that was remote before is no more beyond imagination today; however, it brings about many deleterious effects on older adults' lifestyle. It could be assumed that this planet will have a record number of oldest-old (and centenarians) in the near future. Still, according to Darwinism, there will also be a struggle for existence over a shortage of resources and natural biology, in which younger people will survive and the number of centenarians will decrease dramatically. However, we should be optimistic about how to protect centenarians and their wisdom in the coming years. Alternatively, we may speculate that with the virtue of enjoying better aging, present-day older adults could bring a social revolution by their active social participation to create resources for others who need them. Their guidance on the sustainable lifestyle may impact future generations in a positive way (Bhattacharyya, 2017b).

Although the ancient literature of India uncovers a vast body of resources, the emergence of gerontology as a research domain in India is not satisfactory. It seems we are stuck due to overpopulation and have forgotten our heritage. Currently, there are no significant stand-alone gerontology (degree-level) courses taught in India. Even the term "gerontology" itself is very uncommon in the general population. However, unlike the past years, many scholars at the national and international levels are showing interest in researching aging studies, but more research is necessary to prepare ourselves to provide older adults, more specifically the oldest-old, with the best possible management that would allow them to lead a meaningful life. Rectifying and practicing the factors responsible for maintaining longevity in the general population should be an equal responsibility for every individual, family, society, and the government.

References

Amin, I. (2017). Perceptions of successful aging among older adults in Bangladesh: An exploratory study. *Journal of Cross-Cultural Gerontology, 32*(2), 191–207. https://doi.org/10.1007/s10823-017-9319-3

Barzilai, N., Huffman, D. M., Muzumdar, R. H., & Bartke, A. (2012). The critical role of metabolic pathways in aging. *Diabetes, 61*, 1315–1322.

Bhattacharyya, K. K. (2017a). Health and associated social problems of elderly population in an urban setting: a study from Kolkata, India. *International Journal of Community Medicine and Public Health, 4*(12), 4406–4410.

Bhattacharyya, K. K. (2017b). Centenarians in India: The present scenario. *International Journal of Community Medicine and Public Health, 4*(7), 2219–2225.

Bhattacharyya, K. K., & Molinari, V. (2021). Longevity: Cultural and social influences of a unique non-Western lifestyle. In M. Poulain & J. Mackowicz (Eds.), *Positive ageing and learning from centenarians: Living longer and better* (pp. 111–127). Routledge. Chapter 8, ISBN 9780367753634.

Bhattacharyya, K. K., Hueluer, G., Meng, H., & Hyer, K. (2021a). Movement-based mind-body practices and cognitive function in middle-aged and older adults: Findings from the Midlife in the United States (MIDUS) study. *Complementary Therapies in Medicine, 60*, 102751. https://doi.org/10.1016/j.ctim.2021.102751

Bhattacharyya, K. K., Molinari, V., & Hyer, K. (2021b). Self-reported satisfaction of older adult residents in nursing homes: Development of a conceptual framework. *The Gerontologist*, gnab061. Advance online publication. https://doi.org/10.1093/geront/gnab061

Budovsky, A., Craig, T., Wang, J., Tacutu, R., Csordas, A., Lourenco, J., Freifeld, V. E., & de Magalhaes, J. P. (2013). A database of human genetic variants associated with longevity. *Trends in Genetics, 29*, 559–560.

Buettner. (2012). *The blue zones, second edition: 9 Lessons for living longer from the people who've lived the longest*. National Geographic Society.

Census of India. (2011). *Office of the Registrar General and Census Commissioner, India*. Ministry of Home Affairs, Government of India. Retrieved from: http://www.censusindia.gov.in/2011census/population_enumeration.aspx

Cherry, K. E., Marks, L. D., Benedetto, T., Sullivan, M. C., Barker, A., & for the Louisiana Healthy Aging Study. (2013). Perceptions of longevity and successful aging in very old adults. *Journal of Religion, Spirituality, & Aging, 25*(4). https://doi.org/10.1080/15528030.2013.765368

Dholakia, U. M. (2015). *Why are so many Indian arranged marriages successful? The upsides of relinquishing choice, deciding quickly, & lower expectations*. Psychology Today. Internet source. Retrieved from: https://www.psychologytoday.com/.../why-are-so-many-indian-arranged-marriages-su...

Dionigi, R. A., Horton, S., & Bellamy, J. (2011). Meanings of aging among older Canadian women of varying physical activity levels. *Leisure Sciences, 33*, 402–419. https://doi.org/10.1080/01490400.2011.606779

Evert, J., Lawler, E., Bogan, H., & Perls, T. (2003). Morbidity profiles of centenarians: Survivors, delayers, and escapers. *Journal of Gerontology: Medical Sciences, 58A*(3), 232–237.

Finch, C., & Tanzi, R. E. (1997). Genetics of aging. *Science, 278*(5337), 407–411. https://doi.org/10.1126/science.278.5337.407

Fried, L. P., Ferrucci, L., Darer, J., Williamson, J. D., & Anderson, G. (2004). Untangling the concepts of disability, frailty, and comorbidity: Implications for improved targeting and care. *Journal of Gerontology: Medical Sciences, 59*(3), 255–263.

Govindaraju, D., Atzmon, G., & Barzilai, N. (2015). Genetics, lifestyle and longevity: Lessons from centenarians. *Applied & Translational Genomics, 4*, 23–32. https://doi.org/10.1016/j.atg.2015.01.001

Griffith, R. T. (1899). Chapter 36 Hymn 21 in the *Textbook of White Yajurveda*, pp. 292.

Gupta, B. (2012). *An introduction to Indian philosophy: Perspectives on reality, knowledge and freedom*. Routledge.

Iveniuk, J., Waite, L. J., McClintock, M. K., & Tiedt, A. D. (2014). Marital conflict in older couples: Positivity, personality, and health. *Journal of Marriage and Family, 76*, 130–144.

Kulke, H., & Rothermund, D. (2004). *A history of India* (4th ed., pp. 21–23). Routledge.

Lamb, S. (2014). Permanent personhood or meaningful decline? Toward a critical anthropology of successful aging. *Journal of Aging Studies, 29*, 41–52. https://doi.org/10.1016/j.jaging.2013.12.006

Levenson, R. W., Carstenson, L. L., & Gottman, J. M. (1993). Long-term marriage: Age, gender and satisfaction. *Psychology and Aging, 8*, 301–313.

Nair, M. (2012). Field studies on centenarian experiences in South Asia. *Asian Journal of Gerontology and Geriatrics, 7*, 64.

Passarino, G., Francesco, D. R., & Montesanto, A. (2016). Human longevity: Genetics or Lifestyle? It takes two to tango. *Immunity & Ageing, 13*, 12.

Poulain, M., Herm, A., & Pes, G. (2013). The Blue Zones: Areas of exceptional longevity around the world. *Vienna Yearbook of Population Research, 11*, 87–108.

Radhakrishnan, S. (1962). *Indian philosophy* (Vol. 2). Oxford University Press.

Ramamurti, P. V., & Jamuna, D. (2010). Geropsychology in India. In G. Misra (Ed.), *Psychology in India. Volume 3: Clinical and health psychology* (pp. 185–263). Pearson.

Roser, M. (2017). 'Life Expectancy.' *Published online at* OurWorldInData.org. Retrieved from: https://ourworldindata.org/life-expectancy/ [Online Resource]

Samanta, T., Chen, F., & Vanneman, R. (2015). Living arrangements and health of older adults in India. *The Journals of Gerontology. Series B, Psychological Sciences and Social Sciences, 70*(6), 937–947.

Serra, V., Watson, J., Sinclair, D., & Kneale, D. (2011). Living beyond 100: A report on centenarians. *The International Longevity Centre, UK*. Retrieved from: www.ilcuk.org.uk

Sharma, I., Pandit, B., Pathak, A., & Sharma, R. (2013). Hinduism, marriage and mental illness. *Indian Journal of Psychiatry, 55*(Suppl 2), S243–S249.

Shmerling, R. H. (2018). *The health advantages of marriage.* Harvard Health Blog. Internet source. Retrieved from: https://www.health.harvard.edu/.../the-health-advantages-of-marriage-201611301066...

Tiwari, S. C., & Pandey, N. M. (2013). The Indian concepts of lifestyle and mental health in old age. *Indian Journal of Psychiatry, 55*(Suppl 2), S288–S292.

Vaillant, G. (2002). *Aging well: Surprising guideposts to a happier life from the landmark Harvard study of adult development.* Little, Brown and Company.

Weiss, M. (1986). History of psychiatry in India. *Samiksa, 11*, 31–45.

Xu, M., Thomas, P. A., & Umberson, D. (2015). Marital quality and cognitive limitations in late life. *The Journals of Gerontology. Series B, Psychological Sciences and Social Sciences, 71*(1), 165–176.

Yogananda, P. (1946). *Autobiography of a yogi* (1st ed.). The Philosophical Library (USA). Available at: https://lccn.loc.gov/47000544

Chapter 10
Aging, Disease Prevention, and Technology

10.1 Health Promotion: Nourishing Inner Technologies

In any discussion regarding technology, the first word that comes to mind is "machine." In this perspective, the human body is an amazing and perhaps the most valuable machine that needs to be protected by ourselves.

10.1.1 Hormesis and Aging

Hormesis is an eternal biphasic dose-response physiological mechanism of any biological system, marked by a low dose of stimulation and a high dose of inhibition (Mattson, 2008). On the other hand, aging may be defined as a multicausal progressive failure of maintaining homeostasis in our body. Therefore, there is a huge and unavoidable role of hormesis in human aging. Recently, the concept of hormesis is gaining increased popularity in the field of aging research. Now it is evident that some unavoidable metabolic byproducts like reactive oxygen species (ROS) or reactive nitrogen species (RNS) could act as major mediators of antiaging and neuroprotective processes within a certain concentration window. Therefore, this potential mechanism can be beneficial for health promotion as well as in the direct clinical application. Furthermore, hormesis is proven to be beneficial for age-related morbidities in the domains of calorie restriction, nutrition, radiation, and physical exercise (Rattan & Demirovic, 2009). Therefore, we should keep up our future research to welcome new arenas where hormesis can be applied more to potentially slow the aging process further.

In toxicology, hormesis is a dose-response physiological event, resulting in either a bell-shaped or an inverted U-shaped curve (Bhakta-Guha & Efferth, 2015). Physical exercise induces a similar kind of hormesis curve response in the human

© The Author(s), under exclusive license to Springer Nature Switzerland AG 2021   129
K. K. Bhattacharyya, *Rethinking the Aging Transition*,
https://doi.org/10.1007/978-3-030-88870-1_10

body. Physical activity creates oxidative stress that is dependent on the duration and intensity of the exercise. However, irrespective of reactive oxygen species (ROS) production, physical exercise produces an adaptive response beneficial to many systems of our body. It benefits the nervous system by neurogenesis and producing more neurotrophic factors. It also helps the cardiovascular and musculoskeletal systems by increasing improved oxygenation in cardiac and skeletal muscles, respectively. This process, in turn, affects positive renal and hepatic perfusion. Even in the production of elevated ROS, the bodily systems function in such a manner so that the recovery occurs very quickly. This recovery occurs through ATP regeneration, mainly via glycolytic pathways. Although factors like age and level of fitness may affect the whole process, overall, physical exercise promotes health depending on the adaptive response of the body. Also, regular physical exercise is recommended to prevent a variety of old age morbidities, including Alzheimer's disease.

10.1.2   Hormesis and Calorie Restriction

Everitt and Le Couteur (2007) suggested that the benefit of calorie restriction in humans would be between 3 to 13 years of increased life expectancy. Even though the concluding remarks of Everitt and Le Couteur are just an oversimplification of the fact, still, I think the average benefit would be closer to 13 years. The authors found that being overweight in middle age reduces 3 years from life expectancy, but this number is higher in the case of obese and severely obese participants. These data were collected from different research conducted in different settings with participants of varying age groups. Also, in one study, it is evident that calorie restriction benefits for extremely obese White males are 13 years of increased life expectancy, while in the case of Black males, this number is 20 years. Therefore, the mean should go toward the higher side of the range. Also, the authors expressed the view that regular physical exercise may reduce excess body weight, therefore having an add-on effect. Overall, the claim is very much debatable; still, further longitudinal research outcomes are available.

In the domain of public health, hormesis is a valuable concept where a low dose of a stressor protects against a higher and lethal dose of the same stressor. For example, successive mild myocardial ischemia has a protective role against a sudden myocardial infarction in many cardiac patients. The exposure to least-harmful, minimal doses of amyloid aggregates exerts a protective stimulus from future Alzheimer's disease. Though hormesis describes an evolutionarily beneficial process by which a cell or an entire organism can be preconditioned, we have to keep in mind that any biological system is much more diverse than a machine. One cannot expect an outcome from a biological system only in the way they are thinking. There are a lot more things beyond our knowledge. Therefore, exposures to toxic, lethal, and carcinogenic compounds, however minimal the exposure levels are, may not provide the same health benefits every time. Furthermore, there may be different optimal hormetic windows for different individuals. Therefore, it can be assumed that there is always a chance of misinterpreting hormesis. As a result, researchers should make decisions with an open mind, and their claims must be honest and not only blindly rejecting the thoughts of another.

10.1.3   Cardiovascular Health

Prevention is always better than cure. Therefore, we need to secure the early detection and management of the risk factors that may develop future cardiac morbidities. Many studies suggest a range of behavioral and pharmacologic therapies as positive health promotional factors to defer cardiovascular diseases. The dietary factor is highlighted most often. However, we should take all the modifiable risk factors into account. These include biological risk factors, such as blood pressure, dyslipidemia, endocrinopathy, and obesity, and behavioral risk factors such as physical exercise, addiction, and diet. Also, non-modifiable risk factors like genetic risk factors, age, race, and some infrastructural determinants, such as socioeconomic development and education, play a role in this issue. Therefore, the strategy to postpone the average onset of cardiovascular disease in the population should be based on the collaboration of the best possible and feasible approaches to these determinants.

Some scholars broadened the World Health Organization's definition of health as "a desirable state of complete physical, psychological, social, environmental, and spiritual wellbeing and not merely the absence of disease or infirmity" (Bhattacharyya et al., 2021, p.13). This definition is similar to the concept found in different ancient Indian *Ayurveda* literature. *Yoga*, which was developed in ancient India around the sixth and fifth centuries BCE, is now considered merely a physical exercise in the Western world. However, it is actually a higher conception than that. *Yoga* is a combination of physical, mental, social, environmental, and spiritual practices. Combining the concepts of yoga and Ayurveda in lifestyle modification will possibly yield the best health outcome, not only regarding cardiovascular morbidities but also overall health.

10.1.4   Cognitive Health

At the cellular level, blood glucose concentration directly relates to the circadian pattern of sleep and progressively increases during sleep. As a result, the cells get the required rest and ultimately rejuvenate. With enough sleep, brain cells work much better, their interconnections are restored, and memories are reactivated. This process also helps in creativity, synthesizes new ideas, and helps to maintain cognitive function.

Today's lifestyle demands prolonged wakefulness, which in turn leads to increased tiredness and fatigue. Irregularity in sleep may occur due to lifestyle, shifting duties in the workplace, or traveling across different time zones. Age is probably the most common physiological factor of sleep interruption. Aging disrupts the sleep cycle. Older adults usually spend more time in the lighter stages of sleep than in a deep sleep, though sleep timing may remain unchanged. Sleep disturbance results in multi-organ disturbances. Though the entire pathophysiology is still obscure, many studies suggest that interrupted metabolic functions in brain cells have a negative effect on the proper functioning of different neurotransmitters. Sleep turmoil also leads to increased generation of reactive oxygen species. Long-term persistence of insufficient sleep creates a negative feedback effect on normal brain functioning, specifically cognitive functioning. When this disturbance occurs due to obstructive sleep apnea, it adds a real threat to the development of dementia in later days, particularly when associated with intermittent hypoxemia. Recent studies revealed that obstructive sleep apnea was associated with an earlier age of progression to mild cognitive impairment (MCI) or Alzheimer's disease and Parkinson's disease. Therefore, sleep health has a substantial effect on age-related cognitive decline, directly or indirectly, on a population-wide level.

MCI is one of the possible earlier stages of dementia. There are many overlapping criteria for diagnosing different types of dementia, making it difficult to diagnose even for primary care physicians. Many studies are available, showing the prevalence and the possible consequences of dementia. Still, as there is no definite curative therapy available through the medical model, minimal studies are available showing the direction toward a constructive therapeutic intervention for persons with dementia. Some studies suggest that brain fitness technology (George & Whitehouse, 2011) is a good option. In contrast, some studies suggest MRI scans or other biomarkers as screening techniques (Peterson, 2009) or bi- or multilingualism (Perani et al., 2017) as positive directions, but not enough to gain universal acceptance. We can engage our brains in the same way even in solving day-to-day mathematical puzzles.

However, we have to identify strong and easy ways to move forward. Lifestyle modification is the most important of them. The choice of diet and physical activity is vital for older adults. If they remain physically active on a regular basis, many old-age problems, such as cognitive decline, can be prevented by way of good balance, better blood circulation, and tissue liveness. Engagement with companionship does not require much investment. It is evident that older adults who create intergenerational relationships with children experience substantial health benefits in their quality of living (Bhattacharyya & Molinari, 2021). Here comes the significance of the traditional extended family. This family culture has a big role in longevity and aging well through emotional bonding and discipline. In Indian culture, many children make their best friendship with their grandparents and express themselves without fear of judgment and scolding from them. This relationship is not only an obligation but also is regarded as a necessity in our society. The grandparents, on the one hand, serve the function as an educator, motivator, guide, and companion, and on the other hand, this relation invigorates and energizes older adults, engaging them in various physical and mental activities, which in turn helps to reduce their depression, social isolation, and possible cognitive impairment. Therefore, we do not need to discover new technologies; only self-realization and self-consciousness are enough to minimize possible cognitive decline.

10.1.5   Sensory System

People typically develop vision and hearing problems with advancing age. Visual impairment includes sensitivity to light and difficulty in visualizing distant objects or reading printed materials. On the other hand, hearing problems include difficulty perceiving and differentiating sounds, understanding speech, and auditory processing information.

Current research suggests that neural degeneration is an essential factor for developing future sensorineural hearing loss (Liberman, 2017). This may progress toward various other morbid conditions like tinnitus, balance disorder, and even cognitive impairment and dementia. Also, age-related hearing loss may result in some seriously detrimental effects on cognitive functioning (Guerreiro & Gerven, 2017). Therefore, it seems that vision impairment is more damaging to the quality of life than hearing impairment. If we think about this problem from a different perspective, many adults regularly do their medical checkups for vision, so why do so many people ignore their ears? Maybe, somehow, people think visual impairment is more vital than hearing impairment.

I consider the impacts are not that simple to be generalized. Vision and hearing, both senses, are essential for individuals to interact with the environment, and both are subject to variable amounts of age-related changes. Both cause us great difficulties when they do not work effectively. However, due to the way we use these senses, their losses affect us in different ways. For a painter, the slightest visual loss causes significant difficulties in their performance than hearing loss of equal intensity. Likewise, for a musician, minimal hearing loss can produce considerable damage in his/her capabilities compared to even more significant visual impairment. A psychological factor also plays here. Every organ and sense are vital to us. We feel discomfort in any derangement in any one of them and think that is the most problematic. The impact depends on whether individuals have a visual impairment, hearing impairment, or both and their adaptability to the problem. These are all relative and depend on various sociodemographic factors. The intensity of detrimental effects of sensory losses, either separately or jointly, significantly impacts communication, activities of daily living, socialization, physical activity and safety, independence, and well-being. For older adults, these increase the risk for falls, social isolation, depression, anxiety, and dependence on others accordingly.

10.1.6   *Nutrition*

In my childhood, my grandmother often scolded me for eating sweetened food and beverages. She believed that those foods could destroy our teeth, mind, and heart functions. After growing up, I realized that either many scientists did not have the right concepts, like what my grandmother had, or they were not trustworthy. Therefore, what is the significance of education, science, and technology in our lives? Are all evidence-based claims "deceptive science"? In the present society, every domain is secularized, monetized, and privatized; we are living in a world of confusion. We do not know who the enemy is, what the destroyer is, and which is toxic for us. Therefore, if we consider the so-called claims of science (not the "science") as one of the nutrients, then this is the most important nutrient having an influence on human aging.

"One size does not fit all." Likewise, one food item may not bring about the same beneficial or deleterious health effect on different individuals. It depends on the climate, genetic predisposition, immune status, lifestyle, and many other social determinants of health. *Bhagavad Gita*, the most sacred book in Hinduism, suggests whatever one eats should be in moderation, with utmost gratitude to the food being eaten and to chew and taste it with full satisfaction without rushing for the next thing. The definition of "nutrient" is different in different nomenclature. If we consider "nutrient" as any food item/substance, then I believe the three specific nutrients having the most influence on human aging are sugar, fruit, and turmeric.

10.1.6.1   Sugar

Sugar, more specifically glucose, has a significant impact on almost every system in the human body. Through the $Na^+ K^+$ ATPase pump, glucose enters every cell and even in the brain. Glucose transport protein (GLUT-1) is highly enriched in brain capillary endothelial cells. These transporters carry glucose molecules through the blood-brain barrier. Sugar is essential, but at the same time, it has some negative effects on heart function, cognition, and immune systems, and it accelerates aging with its cumulative negative effects.

10.1.6.2   Fruit

Fruits are beneficial to improve overall health and reduce the risk of morbidities. Fruits are an excellent source of many essential vitamins and minerals, and they are rich in fiber. They are considered tokens of generosity and spirituality. It is considered that there is a strong relationship between fruit and longevity.

10.1.6.3 Turmeric

One of the traditional spices (its extract is known as curcumin) that originated and once was extensively used in India, turmeric is known to be beneficial for a wide variety of diseases and conditions, including those of the skin, pulmonary, and gastrointestinal systems, and pain, wounds, and liver disorders. Turmeric has potent anti-inflammatory, antimicrobial, and anticancer effects. It is also proven to have strong preventative effects against dementia (Amalraj et al., 2016). Water was not considered a nutrient here; otherwise, it must be ranked as the first one.

In the human body, reactive oxygen species (ROS) are formed due to different physiological and pathological processes, and in most cases, these are unavoidable. To cope with this biological mechanism, the process of endogenous antioxidant production already exists. Moreover, the action of different drugs, food, and food supplements is multifaceted. Therefore, the specific pharmacological response of a molecule/compound in the human body largely depends on its source of intake. In the case of antioxidants, this action is still very much debatable. Results of newer research are coming out, which contradict the existing notion regarding antioxidants and their efficacy. These results are disappointing because most of these claims are spurious, misleading, and business-related. Therefore, my opinion is to rely on natural food like fruits, vegetables, and spices that contain enough natural antioxidants to maintain good health rather than trusting in commercially available antioxidant supplements.

10.1.7 Musculoskeletal System

Pain is a protective physiological response of the human body. In older adults, it is a very common phenomenon that has a tremendous impact on the quality of life. Often in clinical practice, our goal is not focused on the complete remission of pain but to reduce its intensity because this directs us toward the diagnosis and thereby to identify the line of management. As the level of tolerance and expression varies significantly from person to person, it is very difficult to create a universally accepted pain assessment tool. In older adults, pain is probably the most underassessed and undertreated symptom. Quality of life largely depends on an individual's physical, psychological, and social health, and in this regard, pain has a massive negative influence on the quality of life.

Musculoskeletal pain is the most common type of pain experienced by older adults. Chronic musculoskeletal pain is associated with various complex biopsychosocial factors that directly affect the quality of life and often require nonpharmacologic interventions to control. *Fibromyalgia* is a chronic problem characterized by pain and tenderness all over the body associated with fatigue, sleep, memory, and mood problems. Fang et al. (2019) evaluated how pain severity through sleep quality affects the cognitive performance of adult fibromyalgia patients. They suggested that better sleep quality can neutralize the adverse effects of pain on cognitive function, thereby improving the quality of life.

Osteoarthritis is a common disease in older adults. It is characterized by the wearing down of the protective tissue layer at the ends of bones, causing joint pain and thereby gradual impairment in physical function, coexisting morbidities, and reduced quality of life. Nonsteroidal anti-inflammatory drugs (NSAIDs), paracetamol, and opioids are the commonly used medications that provide symptomatic relief to osteoarthritis patients. However, long-term consumption of these drugs often causes different adverse effects. Those gastrointestinal, cardiovascular, and renal side effects further cause various comorbidities impacting the quality of life in another way. Tang et al. (2017) found fatigue or tiredness as the most influential factor associated with both daytime and nighttime sleep-related consequences in older adults with comorbid insomnia and osteoarthritis pain. In addition, the authors discussed the implications due to associated psychological distress having a strong negative impact on quality of life. Lee et al. (2017) described how optimizing pain management in patients with osteoarthritis might increase their mobility and participation in physical activity and improve psychosocial engagement.

Research on some alternative approaches also showed promising results. For example, Srivastava et al. (2016) have shown how curcumin, an Indian herb with antioxidant and anti-inflammatory properties, suppresses inflammation and causes clinical improvement in patients with osteoarthritis. The quality of life of osteoarthritis patients will continue to be hampered unless these alternative therapies get widespread acceptance.

10.1.8 Physical Activity

According to the World Health Organization (WHO), "health promotion is the process of enabling people to increase control over, and to improve, their health" (WHO, 1986). Physical activity is one of the health promotion measures, and its promotion requires actions from different levels, such as government, society, and individuals. Awareness is essential for promoting physical activities at the individual level. Physical activity through body movements requires the action of skeletal muscles that need energy expenditure, which can be performed through daily activities, such as walking, playing, carrying out household chores, traveling, and engaging in various recreational activities.

We often confuse the term "physical activity" with "exercise," which is a subcategory of physical activity performed in a planned and organized manner to improve physical fitness. The WHO (2010) suggests older adults should do at least 150 minutes of moderate-intensity physical activity throughout the week, or at least 75 minutes of vigorous-intensity physical activity throughout the week, or an equivalent combination of moderate- and vigorous-intensity activity. Insufficient physical exercise is a modifiable risk factor for different morbidities and mortality.

Physical exercise can be broadly divided into four categories, i.e., endurance, strength, balance, and flexibility. Endurance or aerobic exercise, such as walking or running, is helpful through increased breathing and heart rate. Strength exercise, like resistance training or climbing stairs, is beneficial for health, making our muscles stronger. Balance exercises, such as tai chi and Pilates, help prevent falls, and flexibility exercise, like yoga, stretches muscles. All these activities vary in their components and characteristics but involve multiple organs and improve functions of various bodily systems, such as cardiovascular, musculoskeletal, respiratory, nervous, and endocrine, through different physiological pathways. For example, some researchers suggested that aerobic exercise helps prevent falls, whereas some described resistance training as beneficial for cognitive functioning. All these physical activities overlap in nature, such as yoga, which contains all the components and is beneficial for overall health promotion at any age. Through the aging process, people gradually lose their physical abilities. However, the importance of physical exercise for health and aging may be ranked in the following order: 1) aerobic exercise, 2) stretching, and 3) resistance training.

Yoga, tai chi, and a few other mind-body practices are now considered movement therapies in the Western world. A wide body of research has established that mind-body practices have the potential to influence various physical and psychological characteristics, including cognitive functions (Bhattacharyya et al., 2020; Cramer et al., 2019). On the other hand, both personality traits and cognitive functions are central dimensions of adult behavior and functioning. Future research is essential to study whether personality traits influence an individual's propensity toward mind-body practices as an effective alternative intervention for age-related cognitive decline in older adults. Future research could guide how personality dispositions may protect us from cognitive declines through alternative and complementary practices.

10.1.9   Stress and Behavioral Modifications

The cybernetic theory of stress, coping, and well-being defines "stress" as the negatively perceived discrepancy between the perceived and desired situations functioning in an individual's life (Lavretsky & Newhouse, 2012). During stress, different brain regions, such as the hippocampus, amygdala, and prefrontal cortex, change structurally at the molecular level, shaping our physiological, behavioral, and social responses. When individuals are exposed to a stressor, their sympathetic nervous system is triggered, regulating their gene expression. Consequently, a nuclear factor, kappa B (NF-kB), and cytokines are released that cause inflammation at the cellular level. As a result, a short-lived fight-or-flight reaction may occur, which in turn may produce a beneficial effect. Still, if this remains persistent, it leads to a higher risk of health problems, even accelerating the aging process. Stress is often psychological and associated with daily activities in our modern lifestyle, unlike other animals, where stress is usually associated with life-or-death situations. The process of our gene expression, followed by inflammation, often remains persistent and causes various physical and mental morbidities.

New behavioral interventions are gaining popularity to improve brain functioning and thereby ameliorate chronic stress. Hormesis plays a significant role here. Miller et al. (2017) discussed how physiological adaptation to stress is vital to slow the aging process. Different approaches through calorie restriction, exercise, resilience training, and hormone replacement therapies are showing positive directions. Changing our dietary pattern, avoiding addictions, having adequate rest or breaks from work, and modifying sleep hygiene can bring about dramatic changes in our lives. Individuals who practice mind-body interventions, such as yoga, meditation, and tai chi, show decreased production of NF-kB and cytokines, which opposes the pro-inflammatory gene expression process, thereby decreasing the risk of inflammation-related disorders. Mind-body interventions reduce the level of perceived stress, which consequently improves our well-being in later life.

10.2 Assistive Outer Technologies in Aging

For most of us, only maintaining our "machine" through health promotion is not enough. We need some technologies from the outside to achieve better living. Though we are using technologies in our day-to-day lifestyle, they are still not universally available. Usage of technologies varies from country to country, from society to society, and even from person to person. We have huge curiosity and expectations about how the technology will assist older adults in the coming years. Aging well, in many ways, depends on how we adapt to technological advancement, secure ourselves from climate change, and control over international demographics. The evolution from cash and cryptocurrencies toward a universal means of exchange is gaining popularity day by day so that older adults do not have to manage cash/ cards regularly. Driverless vehicles will likely become the regular mode of transport in the near future. Development in 3D printing has pushed our advancement remarkably. The availability of 3D printers, which are capable of printing human organs, is going to reduce human mortality drastically. Regenerative medicine technology is going to be the mainstream soon. It will provide patients with various lifesaving body parts for replacement, thereby adding more years of life even in late older adulthood. On the other hand, artificial intelligence (AI), with its strong impact in literally every area of our lives, such as education, economy, and healthcare, is going to be more indispensable. Virtual reality will be used instead of "real" reality. It seems like the concept of artificial meat is a little unrealistic today, but it will probably become a more widely used food resource in the coming two or three decades. In vitro cloned meat or lab-grown meat (growing muscle cells in a nutrient serum and encouraging their development into muscle-like fibers) could be another future solution to our food supply problems.

Our growing interest in technology continuously pushes our willingness to invest in these enormous expectations from technology, which gradually becomes a necessity and obligation in our lives. CCTV cameras and their application in long-distance caregiving and to rectify older adult abuse are now a common practice. Sleep and other activity trackers, mood (and sleep)-boosting devices, and smart companions are now new technologies for a large number of populations. GPS trackers in cars, even GPS smart soles, are now used widely. Liftwares are now used to compensate for its user's shaking hand in many diseases like Parkinson's disorders. As older adult generations are transitioning to smartphones, several newer apps are being generated, and these apps are offering them different necessary services in just a click. Amazon Echo is a new device used to interact with and control household appliances, such as lights, fans, and many other gadgets. This is also capable of playing the music of choice. Older adults with mobility problems are now using stairlifts to get around their homes more easily. Smartness is in our kitchen, in our bathroom, and in our bedroom, on such a level that our houses are no longer ordinary, as a whole, turned into "smart homes." More and more activities of our daily lives will be assisted by automation and artificial intelligence in the coming years. Many robotics companies are now working on the development of AI-powered robots that will manage our daily lives. These robots may control the activities of daily living of older adults, relieving the gradually increasing pressures from their family members and the healthcare system.

Keeping all these possibilities in mind, we must say that the majority of older adults across the world is not enjoying the benefits of technological advancement to date. On the other hand, we should also be prepared for the day when technology will become a more significant part of our lives and security concerns will grow. Cyberattacks may increase. In the emergence of smart city concepts, what will be the fate of older adult's autonomy? And their collectivity? We are ruining our next generation's lives, rushing toward technologies. They will suffer from human-induced weather changes in the near future. Scientists have warned that extreme climate is soon going to prevail; we need to be prepared for frequent incidents of hurricanes, tsunamis, floods, and many other natural disasters. Another possible adverse effect that we are going to face is the resistance to antibiotics. The WHO slogan of the "end of antibiotics" is going to hit us from a completely different perspective in the near future. With the gradual rising trend of technology dependence, the employment pattern will be changed entirely. There may be a chance of total reshaping of power dynamics. However, the resources will be the same. Therefore, older adults will have to "struggle for existence" with people in lower age groups. As a consequence, technology dependence may counteract globalization and human mass migration. Technology has created complex health dilemmas spawning bio-ethical analysis among many of us. Perhaps we do not have the answers for the associated ethical issues, such as euthanasia and elder abuse, directly or indirectly.

For instance, we do not have a complete picture of dementia. However, we are already capable of creating dementia villages, not only in the Netherlands (Hogeweyk, the first dementia village in the world) but also in many other countries. The concept is to present persons with dementia with their world, to provide them with full freedom in their life under supervision. This entire world contains a post office, supermarket, grocery, bakery, parks, and many other recreational and necessary places exclusively for persons with dementia. We have recreated their world with various assisted technologies, in and outside their apartments. We are smart to design a supermarket where persons with dementia can buy different commodities with/without paying for them, standing opposite to a nonfunctioning machine (screen). Our idea is great! We assume that they cannot rectify our smartness of showing dignity to them. But what if they can rectify this? We never tried to think from that perspective. Why are they morose? Why do they feel neglected? Why have they become apathetic? And why do they feel insecure? What will happen if they identify our treachery? They will feel more lonely, they will feel more bored, and they will feel more helpless. Their second childishness was confined. They desperately need help and we cannot avoid our responsibilities.

10.3   Uncovering the Technology Within

Common behavioral and psychological strategies are engaging persons with dementia with validation therapy, reminiscence therapy, music therapy, pet therapy, and other meaningful activities (Scales et al., 2018). Dr. William H. Thomas introduced the "alternative joy practice," espoused by the Eden Alternative model, to engage older adults in different meaningful and spontaneous activities in the institutional setting (Thomas, 1996), engaging older adults in gardening and engaging them with animals and birds. But are these not short-lived? After some time, our inner self asks for more technologies. However, at this point, I would like to ask what type of technology are we looking for? When our ancestors discovered a "wheel," was that not technology? When was that "wheel" transformed into a "sun clock" (Konark temple, Odisha, India) and was that not technology? The discovery of stone weapons, the discovery of fire, the discovery of scripts, the discovery of spectacles, the discovery of the first antibiotic, the discovery of radio waves, and the discovery of yoga, everywhere was technology. Technology means closeness not a barrier. A smartphone engulfs our time from various other responsibilities; is that technology? Therefore, what is that technology that creates bondage? It is the "love" for a companion, a long-lasting responsibility. I would love to introduce a new model of long-lasting responsibility with the association of *3Es*: "engagement," "environment," and "exercise." Yoga has the potency to combine these. This bondage is the "technology within" (as shown in Fig. 10.1).

10.4   Conclusion

In Sanskrit, yoga means to add. Yoga is the bondage. The term can be used as the bondage between two generations, the orphan adult and the orphan child. It is evident that physical and social deprivation in early childhood affects psychological development, which impacts cognition in early adolescence. In a longitudinal study

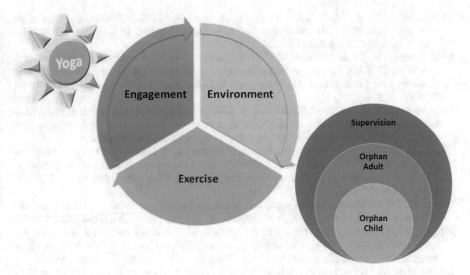

Fig. 10.1 Technology within—a conceptual 3E model for orphan world

(the English and Romanian adoptees study), Beckett et al. (2006) found that very extreme early deprivation factors, such as severe poverty and social exclusion, play a significant role on the impact of the length of and specific psychological development in the early years of life. There were persistent effects of deprivation on cognitive development even in early adolescence. On the other hand, if we just look at our surroundings, we could find numerous older adults feeling lonely and helpless. Assume that if we were to hand over one orphan child to one orphan older adult under supervision, then we can help both to get a new meaning in their lives. This step will be our best expression to show dignity to them. Let us consider our surrounding environment is a big orphan village, where the concerned older adults and the children will practice yoga (as their lifestyle) in addition to their other responsibilities; this will be the ideal technology for humankind. In the next two or three decades, there will be no more orphans in the world.

References

Amalraj, A., Pius, A., Gopi, S., & Gopi, S. (2016). Biological activities of curcuminoids, other biomolecules from turmeric and their derivatives – A review. *Journal of Traditional and Complementary Medicine, 7*(2), 205–233. https://doi.org/10.1016/j.jtcme.2016.05.005

Beckett, C., Maughan, B., Rutter, M., Castle, J., Colvert, E., Groothues, C., Kreppner, J., Stevens, S., O'connor, T. G., & Sonuga-Barke, E. J. (2006). Do the effects of early severe deprivation on cognition persist into early adolescence? Findings from the English and Romanian adoptees study. *Child Development, 77*(3), 696–711.

Bhakta-Guha, D., & Efferth, T. (2015). Hormesis: Decoding two sides of the same coin. *Pharmaceuticals (Basel, Switzerland), 8*(4), 865–883. https://doi.org/10.3390/ph8040865

Bhattacharyya, K. K., Hueluer, G., Meng, H., & Hyer, K. (2020). Mind-body practices in U.S. adults: Prevalence and correlates. *Complementary Therapies in Medicine, 52*, 102501. https://doi.org/10.1016/j.ctim.2020.102501

Bhattacharyya, K. K., & Molinari, V. (2021). Longevity: Cultural and social influences of a unique non-Western lifestyle. In M. Poulain and J. Mackowicz's (Eds.), *Positive Ageing and Learning from Centenarians: Living Longer and Better* (pp.111–127). Routledge, UK. ISBN 9780367753634.

Bhattacharyya, K. K., Molinari, V., & Hyer, K. (2021). Self-reported satisfaction of older adult residents in nursing homes: Development of a conceptual framework. *The Gerontologist*, gnab061. Advance online publication. https://doi.org/10.1093/geront/gnab061

Cramer, H., Quinker, D., Pilkington, K., Mason, H., Adams, J., & Dobos, G. (2019). Associations of yoga practice, health status, and health behavior among yoga practitioners in Germany-Results of a national cross-sectional survey. *Complementary Therapies in Medicine, 42*, 19–26. https://doi.org/10.1016/j.ctim.2018.10.026

Everitt, A. V., & Le Couteur, D. G. (2007). Life extension by calorie restriction in humans. *Annals of the New York Academy of Sciences, 1114*, 428–433. https://doi.org/10.1196/annals.1396.005

Fang, S., Wu, Y., Chen, S., Teng, H., & Tsa, P. (2019). Subjective sleep quality as a mediator in the relationship between pain severity and sustained attention performance in patients with fibromyalgia. *Journal of Sleep Research, 28*(6), e12843. https://doi.org/10.1111/jsr.12843

George, D. R., & Whitehouse, P. J. (2011). Marketplace of memory: what the brain fitness technology industry says about us and how we can do better. *The Gerontologist, 55*(5), 590–596. https://doi.org/10.1093/geront/gnr042

Guerreiro, M. J. S., & Van Gerven, P. W. M. (2017). Disregarding hearing loss leads to overestimation of age-related cognitive decline. *Neurobiology of Aging, 56*, 180–189.

Lavretsky, H., & Newhouse, P. A. (2012). Stress, inflammation, and aging. *The American Journal of Geriatric Psychiatry, 20*(9), 729–733. https://doi.org/10.1097/JGP.0b013e31826573cf

Lee, K., Cooke, J., Cooper, G., & Shield, A. (2017). Move it or lose it. Is it reasonable for older adults with osteoarthritis to continue to use paracetamol in order to maintain physical activity? *Drugs and Aging, 34*, 417–423. https://doi.org/10.1007/s40266-017-0450-1

Liberman, M. C. (2017). Noise-induced and age-related hearing loss: new perspectives and potential therapies. *F1000Research, 6*, 927. https://doi.org/10.12688/f1000research.11310.1

Mattson, M. P. (2008). Hormesis defined. *Ageing Research Reviews, 7*(1), 1–7. https://doi.org/10.1016/j.arr.2007.08.007

Miller, B. F., Seals, D. R., & Hamilton, K. L. (2017). A viewpoint on considering physiological principles to study stress resistance and resilience with aging. *Ageing Research Reviews, 38*, 1–5.

Perani, D., Farsad, M., Ballarini, T., Lubian, F., Malpetti, M., Fracchetti, A., Magnani, G., March, A., & Abutalebi, J. (2017). The impact of bilingualism on brain reserve and metabolic connectivity in Alzheimer's dementia. *Proceedings of the National Academy of Sciences of the United States of America, 114*(7), 1690–1695. https://doi.org/10.1073/pnas.1610909114

Petersen, R. C. (2009). Early diagnosis of Alzheimer's disease: is MCI too late? *Current Alzheimer Research, 6*(4), 324–330. https://doi.org/10.2174/156720509788929237

Rattan, S. I., & Demirovic, D. (2009). Hormesis can and does work in humans. *Dose-Response, 8*(1), 58–63. https://doi.org/10.2203/dose-response.09-041.Rattan

Scales, K., Zimmerman, S., & Miller, S. J. (2018). Evidence-based nonpharmacological practices to address behavioral and psychological symptoms of dementia. *The Gerontologist, 58*(suppl_1), S88–S102. https://doi.org/10.1093/geront/gnx167

Srivastava, S., Saksena, A. K., Khattri, S., Kumar, S., & Dagur, R. S. (2016). Curcuma longa extract reduces inflammatory and oxidative stress biomarkers in osteoarthritis of knee: A four-month, double-blind, randomized, placebo-controlled trial. *Inflammopharmacology, 24*(6), 377–388.

Tang, H. J., McCurry, S. M., Pike, K. C., Von Korff, M., & Vitiello, M. V. (2017). Differential predictors of nighttime and daytime sleep complaints in older adults with comorbid insomnia and osteoarthritis pain. *Journal of Psychosomatic Research, 100*, 22–28. https://doi.org/10.1016/j.jpsychores.2017.06.020

Thomas, W. H. (1996). *Life worth living: How someone you love can still enjoy life in a nursing home: The Eden alternative in action*. Vander Wyk & Burnham.

World Health Organization. (1986). The Ottawa Charter for health promotion: 1st International Conference on Health Promotion. 1986 Ottawa, Canada 17–21 November. Accessed on July 13, 2021, from: https://www.who.int/teams/health-promotion/enhanced-wellbeing/first-global-conference

World Health Organization. (2010). Geneva: World Health Organization. *Global Recommendations on Physical Activity for Health* [Internet]. Accessed on July 13, 2021, from: http://whqlibdoc.who.int/publications/2010/9789241599979_eng.pdf

Chapter 11
Aging and Death

11.1 Death: A Universal Truth

Death is neither an exclusive personal experience nor an event of a particular family; instead, it is a universal truth. Death is one of the two major life events (the other is birth) that is inevitable for all of us, and somehow, we experience it very closely in our lives. I often wonder why death is so impactful in our life. Is it only due to our love for the concerned individual who just passed away? Or is it due to the loss of those things we are accustomed to getting from that individual? This desire may be money, power, love, or any other thing that is important to us. How long should we mourn? When we get an alternative, should we still mourn? Or is it only a temporary hormonal expression? How does it change our future life? I do not know. I saw my paternal grandmother, the late Mrs. Renubala Bhattacharyya, become extroverted and totally different in her lifestyle after the consecutive deaths of her first and second sons, and then husband (my grandfather) after that, in her 40s. I do not know exactly how my grandmother was in her childhood or before marriage. Still, the image I carry of my grandmother is broad-minded, friendly, super energetic, and calculative with a sharp memory. My cousins often mocked her as having a similar brain configuration as one of our former prime ministers. She could remember the names of all her relatives, friends, their dates of births, and even telephone numbers. I have never seen my parents remember all those things, even I cannot remember them. I never saw her scolding any of her grandchildren. She was self-dependent on her widow pension. But I do not know how she perceived the deaths of her three closest ones. Was the outlook of my grandmother a deliberate distraction?

Death is such a natural phenomenon that any death cannot stop other lives instantly; instead, people find ways to substitute the loss and reestablish interest in life. However, some deaths may cause disruption in psychological and physiological functioning for an abnormal period to the close ones of those who have passed. Often this shows some cultural variations. Some individuals may need support for grief after the death of their loved ones. This support may be informal (family support) or formal (treatment). Interpersonal therapy, often with cognitive-behavioral therapy, is the commonly used treatment strategy to cope with the trauma associated with the death and facilitate the mourning process. According to the famous psychologist Robert Neimeyer, the grieving process is not as simple as it is presently thought and depends on a multitude of factors. An individual's life story is fundamental when it comes to an understanding of how they will grieve, particularly the association of their story in relation to the person who has passed. According to Neimeyer, the bereavement pattern is like rewriting individuals' life stories, where some people might play a central part when they were alive but no longer continue to play that role after their death. Rebuilding of life and finding its meaning after someone's death is essential for their close ones. If someone knows for a longer period of time that their loved one is passing, the situation is easier to manage than a sudden or unexpected death. If someone has a long-continued illness and has been suffering for years, their death may give a feeling that they do not have to suffer anymore. The number of days in the dying process is crucial, and in an unexpected death, it is much harder for the close ones as they were not prepared for their loved one's sudden passing.

Even after reading the book *Hospital Land USA* many times, I was still confused about how to describe the feelings of the author (Simonds, 2017). I do not know if the author will agree with me or not; still, in my opinion, the author wanted to become distracted from the vulnerable environment of the hospital, which compelled her to take distancing strategies from illnesses of her close ones (not individuals). I worked for a long time as a healthcare provider in the "land" of a tertiary care hospital in India. It was overcrowded, dirty, and unhygienic, lower in every parameter than what it should be. The environment was not comparable with "airport" or "university," even in its best possible days. Still, everyone is trying to cope with hospital time, as the author did. Although "it is hard to maintain your sense of humor in medical environments" (Simonds, 2017, p. 5), still people can distract themselves with their own formula: patients with their pain of illness or painful medical procedures, a clinician or paramedic with their rude behavior and busy daily schedule, and patient parties (companion) with their active involvements. These are all protective responses. But the time one becomes free (work-less) in hospital land and the time one gets relieved from any scheduled engagement, a fear of impending death (loss) comes to mind. This feeling is a terrifying situation that I faced so many times. Maybe this was a professional hazard, which influenced me to hide something from the public eye. Perhaps this is why the camera lens is similar to a pathological lens or clinical lens but is always different from a sociological lens.

11.2   Death Education

Death education is quite significant in this respect. In the article "Death Education…," Kellehear (2015) interestingly raised his voice for considering death education as a public health issue. First, the domain of death education is not a small one; instead, it is a multidisciplinary and multidimensional topic involving religious studies, philosophy, social sciences, psychology, history, and even medicine. Second, as people have shallow exposure to death and dying, their knowledge on this subject is also abysmal. Here comes the significance of death education. If it is made a part of compulsory education in the school, work, or play environment, people will be familiar with the subject; they will acquire more knowledge about managing psychological stress associated with dying and death. Indeed, this will be a remarkable step to prevent unnecessary and early death. Every year thousands of people die due to snakebite, of which most of the death occurs due to panic (stress for impending death), not from poisonous venoms. Death is a normal destination for every life on this planet, but we should manage the pre-death situation with a calm mind. This awareness is the ultimate purpose of death education.

11.3   Death: Cultural Perspectives

If we view death from a modern-day perspective, there is a huge transition in individuals' feelings about death. In his book chapter "In Our Hearts Forever," James Green (in *Beyond the Good Death: The Anthropology of Modern Dying*) presented a vivid description of the transition of obituary sentiments from ancient Greek civilization to the present day. His narrative flew smoothly from one point to the next, delineating, in today's life, how all our traditional beliefs and faith experiences are gradually sinking into oblivion. Our cyber technologies even have commercially engulfed the obituary sentiments (Green, 2008). Virtual cemeteries may be safer than the traditional ones in terms of damages from natural causes such as inclement weather; however, are virtual cemeteries bounded with real emotional connections? In my opinion, this is nothing but shameful commercialization of this mundane world. Real cemeteries are also commercial ventures now. I assume that the author also had a hesitation in adopting present materialistic thoughts, as he mentioned the *poiesis* of memory as the modern substitution of soul. However, the existence of the soul is accepted in most cultures. For instance, in Hindu culture, it is believed that the destination of a soul in the astral plane is solely influenced by life activities and the nature of the mind. Often it is also not easy to readjust this transition after death.

   Green (2008) also presented different ancient Greek notions regarding the afterlife and various death rituals. He also described the then social status of women (how they were shown as dependents) and the physical existence of mind and memory in the human body. Every civilization has its unique notions and beliefs. In Hindu cultures (which have a 1500–600-BCE-old history), the mind was defined as *manas*, but it was not that "mind" as defined in modern medical science. It was like a receptacle for the senses where all memories and perceptions are stored and used by intelligence to make decisions. *Manas* stores the latent impressions (*samskaras*), which become part of the casual body at the time of death. It was believed that the memory center is located at *Muladhara*, at the base of the spine. The seven *chakras* are responsible for higher consciousness. Yoga and meditations were advised to control our minds. In ancient Hindu literature, the social status of women was shown differently at different periods. But in most of those books, the entire literature considered details for the male lifestyle only. It was delineated in various literature that a wife followed her husband faithfully in different phases of the life course.

There is an eternal truth that persists in the context of our last meeting with anyone, which is "hesitation." Though individuals may react differently, the uneasiness still remains the same. In our childhood, we used to believe (what our grandparents taught) that a person becomes a star in the sky after death. I still think that a person, after death, goes to another "world" or another "dimension" and can "read" anything. I believe that even if you do not confess anything, reading your emotions, they will know everything after death and may forgive you. Therefore, at least try to be present in those final moments: you do not need to say anything; you only need to confess your words through visual expressions. Dying persons are most generous; most of the time, they forgive everything. But if you react artificially, it will cause more exhaustion for the dying person during their transition.

Every culture has its unique and traditional thoughts in every aspect of life. Although traditional extended family culture is prevalent in India, a great variation exists in different ethnic groups, religions, and regions in several other aspects. Still, as in every domain, the country possesses the phenomenon of "unity in diversity." Death and funerals are also not an exception, and funerals, like weddings and many other rituals, are considered a family affair. To some extent, the trend is similar to North American culture, as friends and relatives are invited to both. Still, in most cases, the dead body is cremated in Indian culture rather than being buried. Also, there is a difference in rituals in how the body is dealt with before cremation. The caste system has a profound influence on the whole process in India. However, the common Hindu belief about cremation is that it releases individuals' spiritual souls from their transient physical body to their rebirth. Moreover, with no expenses for the coffin, burial method, monument, and land (or plot), a cremation cost is much lower than the traditional burial costs (Glass & Samuel, 2011). Currently, in the United States, although burials have been the norm, an increasing number of people are opting for cremation; the rate of cremation rose to 34% in 2007, up from 15% in 1985 (Glass & Samuel, 2011).

On the contrary, Gary Laderman's book chapter "Death During Wartime" (in *The Sacred Remains: American Attitudes Toward Death, 1799–1883*) is a gruesome narration of incidences and aftereffects of the American Civil War (Laderman, 1996). Although the discussion is not for the fainthearted, it is a detailed and pragmatic analysis of a portion of the American funerary system. In my opinion, the author somehow criticized the attitudes of people toward death itself, especially with respect to the physical remains. But at the same time, everything regarding those unorthodox deaths was not in their control by any means. Any war has a tremendous impact not only on those fighting on the battlefield but also on their close ones and those who even do not know them. War shows that individuality has no meaning; everything is controlled by an institution (or authority or country). The recent COVID-19 pandemic has shown how helpless we are in a warlike environment. Our personal opinions, feelings, and moral values are of no importance; everything is politicized during our lifetime and even after death. September 11 is such a tragic incident in the United States that everyone related to it would like to forget. From our country's (India) perspective, I can well imagine the nationwide aftereffects of these kinds of events. While under British rule (until 1947), incidents like the "Jallianwala Bagh massacre" or after the "India-China War, 1962," or the recent "terrorist attacks" in different places of India show how weak an individual is in front of institutional politics. Despite all the brutal violence happening around us, we are improving technologically(!). We are giving birth to the "business of death" and nourishing it, too, irrespective of society, irrespective of country.

11.4   Death: Ethical Issues

There is an emotional description of death in a book chapter by Mary Roach (Roach, 2003). In the last sentence of the chapter, the author raised one of the most controversial topics regarding brain death vs. cardiorespiratory death. Although new devices are practiced nowadays, rigor mortis is still considered a confirmatory sign of death. Brain death is such a sensitive issue; even we, the physicians, often want to avoid this situation. In India, there is no legal definition of death. Section 46 of the Indian Penal Code states, "the word 'death' denotes the death of a human being unless the contrary appears from the context" (Dhanwate, 2014, p. 596). Still, some legal issues exist regarding "brain death" and "brain stem death." As a result, while writing death certificates in India, we still prefer to use the term "cardiorespiratory failure." On the other hand, I feel that the chapter is a kind of awareness about organ donation. With the progression of the "green corridor" as well as our positive minds, we want to increase the number of organ donations without thinking of what happens to our souls. In my opinion, organ donation does not affect the ultimate and posthumous journey of the souls, although I am confused by whether this creates a burden for the soul, at least for some time immediately after death.

"The Discomfort of Doctoring" is another emotional piece of literature (Montross, 2007). This writing is a well-presented and easy-to-read narrative of a physician's feelings that flow smoothly from one experience to another. It was a very emotional reading for me, being a physician, as we (most of us!) always try "to treat our patients (and their bodies, when, in life or death, the humanness of them seems elsewhere or gone) with tenderness and empathy and honor" (Montross, 2007, p. 181). I can well remember my first few days as a medical student in the anatomy hall, where I was dissecting an unknown, formalin (formaldehyde)-soaked cadaver with other unknown or little-known male and female classmates. Still, nobody felt uneasy while handling different body parts. Or, in clinics, as final-year medical students, we (by that time we, the classmates, became close friends) never felt awkward/uneasy while examining even private parts of patients of another gender irrespective of age group. I think this is what we called a "professional mindset" that developed (maybe automatically) on the very first step when we entered medical school, and it drove us toward a professional goal. Our personal feelings, shyness, and emotions are meaningless in front of that achievement. I always try to examine female patients in the presence of another female person (maybe a nurse, patient companion, even the woman at the front desk of my clinics). Still, there were so many occasions when I had to examine female patients without a female attendant (maybe due to unavailability at that time) in acute emergency cases. Every physician/surgeon has to face these types of situations. Our professional ethics direct us to handle the situation, and that is why the doctor-patient relationship is called a noble one. However, present materialistic aggression, greed, and surrounding stress are getting their paws on this relationship in different ways. Therefore, everywhere, we need to raise our voice, as much as possible, to protect this trustworthy relationship.

Palliative care is another sensitive domain and is definitely "a-step-ahead" movement toward the practicability of end-of-life care. In this context, as an autopsy cannot bring back life to the concerned dead body, only a general discussion on palliative care cannot yield any fruitful outcome. When and where to stop even a "burdensome and purposeless treatment" is relative. It varies from country to country, society to society, person to person, and physician to physician. No one, no law, and no country can enforce it. That is why "euthanasia" still has not gained universal acceptance. Even for a nuclear family, it is not easy for all the members to reach a consensus. This situation is one of the most sensitive issues in human life. One phrase that is very commonly used is "doctors are next to God." Doctors can try to prolong the life of patients (even unnecessarily), but as they cannot create life (reproduction is an individual issue, not professional), as a professional, they cannot make decisions for abatement of treatment. So, this endless discussion will continue (maybe forever). "Our ultimate goal, after all, is not a good death but a good life to the very end" (Gawande, 2014, p. 245); still, we need to walk a long way to generate awareness, to get a consensus on that.

11.5   Death and Advance Care Planning

Advance care planning is one of the directives of end-of-life care; it is not just about old age. A medical emergency could leave one unable to make decisions about their own health condition at any age. Irrespective of one's present health condition, healthcare planning for the future is vital to make sure one is obtaining the desired medical care. When one is unable to make decisions, doctors and family members may decide for the person concerned. Dementia is one of the devastating causes of later life turmoil. It not only affects the concerned older adult but also destroys the lives of the persons surrounding them. Although modern medical advancement has a great impact on longevity, its role in enhancing the quality of life remains questionable. Moreover, the prolongation of later life sometimes creates frustration among the informal caregivers. Many healthcare providers and families support palliative care as the best option for advanced dementia (Mitchell et al., 2004). However, a large proportion of persons with dementia had no order of advance directives (Mitchell et al., 2004). This creates multiple problems among residents (including problems in care like pressure ulcers, physical restraint use, and treatment with antipsychotic drugs) and family members. Kale et al. (2016) found that 40% of the National Health and Aging Trends Study (NHATS) participants, who are also Medicare beneficiaries, had not discussed their end-of-life medical care preferences. Therefore, management and educational strategies for all the possible aspects of caregiving should be promoted for end-of-life care in general and a palliative approach in advanced dementia care.

Currently, we are going through an era when there is a trend everywhere that everyone is running around like a maniac. We do not know our destination, but we are still running. We are trying to improve ourselves, our science, and our technology. Modern medicalization is a part of this movement. In most cases, we are prolonging our lives for business purposes, with an emotional impulse on the sensitive issue of decision-making in end-of-life care. Is this necessary? Alternatively, we may speculate that one day, a record number of oldest-old will surround us and our world will have only caregivers and care recipients. We will lose all other interests in life, except caregiving (either formal or informal). Therefore, we have to be prepared for the future. In my opinion, every person should make a "will" (or advance directive) regarding their "death commitment," and it must be done before they reach their 60th year. However, various opinions and counter-opinions exist regarding the systematization of the content, execution, and acceptance of advance care planning (Kale et al., 2016).

Healthcare providers should be encouraged to discuss healthcare planning and advance directives with individuals and their families. Reimbursing physicians for advance care planning is a good option (Kale et al., 2016); however, physicians should take additional responsibility. Raising mass awareness is essential for this sociocultural development in any heterogeneous society; therefore, the ongoing social and political effort of major foundations and from the government should be continued. It is essential to consider the importance of the durable powers of attorney for healthcare. It seems that written documents can only go so far and that to maximize your chances of having decisions made in accordance with your values, you need to have a close relative or friend who knows you very well to assist with the decision-making. It seems written documents can only go so far regarding clear-cut decisions in medical care, which we know are less common than we would like.

I always respect older adults and their wisdom. However, sometimes to protect those unnecessarily, we should not ignore the budding stages of our future generation. Modern medicalization snatches the hope of individuals in many ways. The cost of medicalization ruins many families (at least I know in my country) only for responsibility and emotion. Medicalization should focus on promoting "aging well" by providing "healthy aging" and should not be used for "frustrating adulthood" or "snatching childhood." We all desire our death to come naturally. However, even if it comes naturally, could we protect our loved ones' grieving processes from the overwhelming medicalization? Advance care planning provides us with options to choose, from nursing home therapeutic care to palliative care in a person-centric way; however, honest healthcare delivery is necessary for any option.

11.6   The Final Story

This discussion will remain incomplete if I do not mention the article, "I Know How I Want to Die" by Elena Lister (2001). Although there were no older adults (except grandpa and grandma) in the narration, in my opinion, this is one of the most powerful pieces on death. I do not know how I should describe my feelings. I enjoyed it! I liked it! I loved to read the story of a dying kid! No, never, but I know that I have not even finished reading all 16 pages; I could not and cried after long days; I cannot express my feelings, even in my mother tongue. It took me back to my workplace, the gruesome pediatric leukemia ward, where the parents are not even "lucky" like Elena and Phil, because only mothers can stay with their child due to official rules. Helpless fathers can only meet them during "visiting hours." But they cannot afford the cost of "hospice care," even though it is very uncommon in India. For the long-term chemotherapy period (week after week for different intra- and inter-cycles and after obvious relapses), they have to stay in the "hospital land." One particular bed becomes their only "home," leaving behind their original home where their other children (in most cases), daily life events, and memories remain. Though the only disease that has a 100% mortality rate is "rabies," still, in my opinion, leukemia (specifically acute lymphocytic leukemia or ALL) is the most gruesome disease in the world. It just ruins a family; still, parents spend their every effort with a false hope to get their child back. While reading this article, I just wanted to get out of the house, to go to the middle of nowhere and scream, "would anybody please tell me why I am here (the United States)!"; it would echo and echo; I would hold my head with my hands around it to get relief from that stifling situation and hear a voice from someone invisible, "you left your ground like a coward." Yes, I left, I admit it, but I am helpless; a doctor can do nothing; chemotherapy can do nothing; medicine cannot protect life, cannot protect feelings. I have tried to protect my only son from the heartless professional medicalization. I am not going to prepare these flowers for "bone-marrow transplantation" anymore; I will not do "lumbar puncture" on these flowers anymore; I am not going to add any extra painful days to their lives; I cannot withstand the stress anymore; I just want to leave my profession. I am searching for that calmness and maturity that a 6-year-old girl, Liza, had and that probably all 4-, 5-, 6-, and 7-year-old leukemia patients have. Liza and your friends, anywhere you go after death, stay blissful. God will bless you.

References

Dhanwate, A. D. (2014). Brainstem death: A comprehensive review in Indian perspective. *Indian Journal of Critical Care Medicine, 18*(9), 596–605. https://doi.org/10.4103/0972-5229.140151

Gawande, A. (2014). *Being mortal: Medicine and what matters most in the end.* Metropolitan Press. ISBN: 978-1410478122.

Glass, A. P., & Samuel, L. F. (2011). A comparison of attitudes about cremation among Black and White middle-aged and older adults. *Journal of Gerontological Social Work, 54*(4), 372–389. https://doi.org/10.1080/01634372.2010.544379

Green, J. W. (2008). In our hearts forever. In *Beyond the good death: The anthropology of modern dying* (pp. 152–186). University of Pennsylvania Press.

Kale, M. S., Ornstein, K. A., Smith, C. B., & Kelley, A. S. (2016). End-of-life discussions with older adults. *Journal of the American Geriatrics Society, 64*(10), 1962–1967. https://doi.org/10.1111/jgs.14285

Kellehear, A. (2015). Death education as a public health issue. In Stillion & Attig (Eds.), *Death, dying, and bereavement* (pp. 222–232). Springer.

Laderman, G. (1996). Death during wartime. In *The sacred remains: American attitudes toward death, 1799–1883* (pp. 96–116). Yale University Press.

Lister, E. (2001). I know how I want to die. In *Giving a voice to sorrow: Personal responses to death and mourning.* Steve Zeitlin and Ilina Harlow, eds. (pp. 120-134). : Perigree.

Mitchell, S. L., Kiely, D. K., & Hamel, M. B. (2004). Dying with advanced dementia in the nursing home. *Archives of Internal Medicine, 164*(3), 321–326. https://doi.org/10.1001/archinte.164.3.321

Montross, C. (2007). The discomfort of doctoring. In *Body of work: Meditations on mortality from the human anatomy lab.* Penguin.

Roach, M. (2003). How to know if you're dead: Beating-heart cadavers, live burial, and the scientific search for the soul. In *Stiff: The curious lives of human cadavers* (pp. 167–198). WW Norton.

Simonds, W. (2017). *Hospital land USA: Sociological adventures in medicalization.* Routledge.

Chapter 12
Aging and Spirituality

12.1 Hinduism: The Sacred Journey of the Soul, in Life and Afterlife

Om Bhur-Bhuvah Svah
Tat-Savitur-Varennyam |
Bhargo Devasya Dhiimahi
Dhiyo Yo Nah Pracodayaat ||

The *Gayatri Mantra*, the sacred hymns of Hinduism, was created and first enchanted probably many thousands of years ago, chronicled in the ancient Indian scripture *RigVeda* (10:16:3) (Rajhans, 2018). I have been chanting this mantra regularly since my sacred thread ceremony ("Upanayana") over 30 years ago. However, with the progression of time, I feel that I have gradually realized its significance. Many people have interpreted its meaning in their own way. In my realization, "OM" is the sacred hymn that is spread throughout everywhere, across the physical plane, spaces, or astral plane and in the consciousness of our spiritual entity, the sacred glow that is most adored for everyone; I meditate that supreme power to awaken my spiritual beliefs.

We have achieved many things due to technological advancements and globalization, which were imagined just a decade ago. However, are we satisfied with our lives, with our achievements? Much confusion clouds our vision in this turmoil. Positive spirituality may be a way of life in the present circumstances, and Hinduism, the ancient Indian tradition, would be a good option. Regarding the all-around development of an individual, India's societal and spiritual concept is still underrepresented in the Western world. My recent propensity toward aging studies has further increased my desire to relate my spiritual beliefs with the idea of the soul. From this perception, I have tried to discover the ideal and satisfactory way of lifestyle. While exploring literature on the sacred journey of the soul, both in life and the afterlife, I have entered more deeply into different concepts of Hinduism and

155
K. K. Bhattacharyya, *Rethinking the Aging Transition*,
https://doi.org/10.1007/978-3-030-88870-1_12

found a heavenly pleasure. I have also found the influence of Hinduism on other ancient civilizations, notably Aztec, Mayan, and Inca cultures, while doing a comparative study. Being a geriatric physician and from a continuous dealing with older adults in India, I often wondered about how most of these individuals keep their positive outlook alive, especially regarding death. I realized that the big five personality traits are nothing but the *sattvic*, *rajasic*, and *tamasic gunas* described in different Hindu texts and I have a strong relationship with this outlook. These feelings also inspired me to search for the possible answers to one of the eternal questions, i.e., is the idea of souls a pragmatic one, and if so, then why are they (the souls) wandering?

12.2   Concepts of Soul and Reincarnation in Hinduism

Death is neither an exclusive personal experience nor an event of a particular family; instead, it is a universal truth. Death is one of the two major life events (the other is birth) that is inevitable for all of us, and somehow we all experience it very closely in our lives. Although the knowledge regarding death and the afterlife is not limited to any specific culture, it still cannot be complete without a discussion of ancient literature of the Eastern culture, especially Hinduism. It is probably the oldest living religion in the world with a history of thousands of years. Although the specific notion of the afterlife shows considerable variation in different cultures and ethnic groups, the ultimate concept regarding the posthumous journey of the soul is similarly depicted almost everywhere (Grof, 2010).

The *soul* is a common term used to denote our self-conscious life force. A living soul is considered one's self-conscious life force with the sense of "I" (Abhedananda, 1944). This realization of "I" unifies everything together and creates a smooth harmony in every step of our life. For example, an orchestra may be decorated with different instruments. Still, each device needs to be played in its own but in a synchronized manner, following its conductor's direction, to produce harmony. Similarly, as organs of our body continue functioning in a coordinated way, it also creates harmony. Now, who is the conductor of the organs in our body? This director is invisible in the eyes of orthodox science, but advanced science tells us about that director, who has absolute control over the whole-body system (Abhedananda, 1944). Here comes the concept of the soul, which leaves our body just after death (Abhedananda, 1944).

The concept of heaven and paradise also varies in different cultures and religions (Grof, 2010). According to Hinduism, heaven and hell are the conceptions of our minds. Technically these are not present in the real world. In the journey of the soul (including our life course when the soul becomes an integral part of our mind), it has to pass through different states. We experience all these, until we belong to the condition of ignorance. However, once we realize our real existence with the absolute spirit, we become free from mundane concepts like birth and death. At this point, our actuality reaches its purest state and reigns in its magnificence of eternity

(Bhagavad Gita, Chap. 2, Verse 27). Hindu philosophy delineates that our soul is divine in the purest sense of the word. It is nothing but our past activities ("karma") that are responsible for its bondage with mundane matters; the soul attains its perfection only when this earthly bond gets destroyed, and subsequently "Moksha" (or "Mukti," freeness) is achieved. It is the ultimate freedom from the bonds of death and incarnation (Vivekananda, undated). "Dharma" is the mediator or counteracting linkage between *karma* and *moksha*. *Dharma* is the righteous way to lead our lives. According to Dr. Bina Gupta, "*Dharma* as a system of rules governs every aspect of human life in the human's relationship to himself, to his family, to his community, to the state, to the cosmos, and so on" (Gupta, 2012, p. 12).

Vedanta philosophy, a lineage of Hindu philosophy, is strongly based on the concepts of mortality and reincarnation. It suggests that if anything has birth, it must die; consequently, anything that is dead must retake birth (Abhedananda, 1944). Hinduism does not believe that the soul is created by God or by any other supernatural being. It is considered that a soul is neither born nor dead. The soul is an eternal and immortal entity and can take any form it likes to take (Abhedananda, 1944). It is assumed that our individual lives are only a part of numerous waves of an infinite ocean, which are moving forward endlessly. Individuals design their destination invariably; we build our past, present, and future through our activities (*karma*) (Abhedananda, 1944, p. 54). The theory of Hinduism does not believe in the destruction of everything by death; it thinks that death is a transition of the body (Bhagavad Gita, chapter 2.20, & Katha Upanishad, chapter 1.2.18). This transition is just like the transformation of energy, which remains the same. Vedanta philosophy teaches that the circumference of every soul is an infinite one, centering a particular body, and after death, this center shifts from one body to a different one (Vivekananda, undated). The soul only changes the cloth from the older one to a newer one. This transition of the soul is believed to happen in three stages. First, the soul departs the old body through one of the nine different holes (two eyes, two ears, two nostrils, mouth, and two excretory orifices) present in our body. Then the soul travels to the location of its next body and ultimately finds a new body (The Brihadaranyaka Upanishad, chapter 4.4.122). This intermediate stage is painful for the soul (the soul in this phase is called "Preta"). For this reason, certain rituals are performed by the relatives of the concerned person (as per Hindu Shastra) to make this journey as smooth as possible. In the last phase, the soul enters the womb of a mother to continue its mission. The point through which the soul departs the previous body indicates its next destination. This departure is determined by the desire and activities (*karma*) of the concerned soul in the past (Bhagavad Gita, chapter 15.8).

The concept of Hinduism was formed through a kind of revelation called the "Vedas." The Hindus hold the belief that the *Vedas* neither have any beginning nor end. It may be unusual to hear that a book has neither a beginning nor an end. Indeed, the word *Vedas* does not point to any specific book. It is the accumulated treasury of spiritual knowledge expressed by many erudite individuals at different times that are recorded in various pieces of ancient Hindu literature (Vivekananda, undated). Many yogis and sages (also known as "Rishis," many of whom were women) nurtured all these thoughts in ancient ages. Although at that time there were no books, the textual materials were heard and verbally transmitted by the earthly sages from generation to generation and called "Shruti"/"Smriti" (as everyone only remembered the knowledge). This sacred literature comprising four *Vedas* (*Rig*, *Saam*, *Jajur*, and *Atharva*), along with *Brahmanas* (ritual practices), *Aranyaka* (forest books), and *Upanishad* (philosophical details), is collectively called the "Vedas" (Van Buitenen, 1998).

Vedanta philosophy reveals that the universe consists of matter/object and mind/soul in equal proportion, which cannot be separated. What we think or feel in our everyday life cannot be produced through any mechanical processes (Abhedananda, 1944). Modern science says that motion can only produce motion. Then how can these atomic motions produce consciousness in our body? There must be some other causative agents behind this that are different from the nuclear concept. This concept is *the soul*. Knowledge of matter is the perception of our mind through which we are consciously doing our mundane activities. Beyond this, we can only imagine but don't know exactly. Our mind cannot go beyond itself. With our earthly bodies, we are now living in three dimensions. After death, the soul leaves this three-dimensional physical plane and goes to another plane. This plane is beyond our conceptional framing of the materialistic world. This place exists in the fourth dimension, where the souls rest after leaving their physical world (Abhedananda, 1944). Life after death means the continuity of life in this apparent imaginary world.

According to Hinduism, in the persistent reincarnation process, a soul needs to go through many cycles of birth and death in order to enter a different body. Through this process, eventually, it reaches the perfection to achieve freeness (*Mukti* or *moksha*) toward the ultimate status (Abhedananda, 1944). During the progression to a higher status, our ancient yogis practiced "Samadhi" in different forms, and any *Samadhi* is superior to "death" in the concept of bringing one (the sages) to a divine state, the ultimate control of the life force and mind. It is a complete harmony, when the controlled mind unites with the soul ("Atma") (Abhedananda, 1944) like a solution. In the fundamental language of physics, "quantum" denotes the minimum quantity of energy involved in an interaction; when this energy bursts, they collectively form the cosmos. Our internal structure is also formed by the same energy, our life force. Seven ultrafine bodies hold different forms of information, and they resemble the "chakra system." These layers are "the etheric body (first layer), the emotional body (second layer), the mental body (third layer), the astral level (fourth layer), the etheric template body (fifth layer), the celestial body (sixth layer), and the causal body or ketheric template (seventh layer)" (Lucas, 2014). By simply meditating with single-mindedness through a true meditative practice like yoga, one can accomplish their universality, but it's actually not that "simple" or easy. The great Indian yogis often accomplished this; however, many true yogis have been misunderstood as a lunatic (*Unmad*) by the general population because of their unnatural behavior in a materialistic world.

12.3 The Concept of God in Hinduism

From the perspective of religion, every religion worships certain gods. Still, there are contradictions, and we are fighting to protect our thoughts. Hinduism teaches us that all these thoughts, as well as contradictions, are apparent. The contradictions are only due to adapting the same truth in varying natures (Vivekananda, undated). If we imagine a concept of universal religion, it must be infinite. The same God will bless the followers of all religions, both innocents and evildoers, in the same intensity. This relation will discover holiness in every individual irrespective of age, gender, habitat, social status, and time frame; the blessings will collectively create humanity to realize its truth, its spiritual nature (Vivekananda, undated).

Because of the presence of many gods and goddesses, Hinduism is often considered polytheistic (Greek *poli* means "many" and *theos* means "god"). A notion exists in the general population that Hinduism considers the existence of 33 crore (3.3 billion) gods. However, this is entirely a misconception. Ancient Hindu literature considered "trayastrimsati koti," i.e., 33 *koti* (in Sanskrit, *koti* means "type") or types of gods (Das, 2019); later, it was mistranslated and became synonymous with 33 crore gods. Vedas depicted 33 types of gods as 8 *Vasus*, 11 *Rudras*, 12 *Adityas*, 1 *Indra*, and 1 *Prajapati* (The Brihadaranyaka Upanishad, chapter 1.9.2). The 8 *Vasus* are earth, water, fire, air, ether, moon, sun, and star; the 11 *Rudras* are Praana, Apaana, Vyaana, Samaana, Udaana, Naag, Kurma, Krikal, Devadutta, and Dhananjaya (the ten *Pranas*) and the human soul; each of the 12 months is considered as *Aditya*; *Indra* is the great force of electricity; and *Prajapati* or *Yajna* is the power of purification (Ninan, 2008; WordZz, 2021).

Many Western philosophers consider polytheism as an inferior belief system to monotheism (Greek *mono* means "single") (Fowler, 2002, pp. 22–24). However, with its subtle concept and deeper philosophical meaning, Hinduism always acknowledges the unified Brahman, where all deities are one. Furthermore, "Within material existence, Brahman is said to manifest as the trinity that comprises Brahma, who is the creator of the visible universe; Vishnu, who is the preserver of this creation; and Shiva, who is the agent of change and movement" (Fontana, 1999, p. 96). Western theism almost invariably believes in the separate existence of God and nature. In this respect, many critics regard Hinduism as pantheistic (Greek *pan* means "total/entire"), which considers everything is God. Whatever the terminology is, all of these are created with very limited human knowledge, without knowing the absolute reality. This concept is an unnecessary attempt to confine the infinite into our materialistic wisdom. Hindu philosophy is a much greater concept; it has had a definite impact on other religious beliefs from year after year. Since years back, these apparent belief systems in Indian culture helped to form the unique, diverse, vivid, and peaceful camaraderie.

12.4   Influence of Hinduism on the Societal Structure of India

In the present day, everyone wants to proclaim superiority by directing others, but no one is ready to follow those directions. Here comes the significance of the Indian traditional societal concept. As mentioned earlier, in Hinduism, the marital relationship is considered one of the most important for aging well. In Hinduism, marriage is regarded as the relationship of souls, which extends beyond a single life through incarnations. In Hinduism, spirituality, along with its clinical implication, is prioritized as a more inclusive concept than religion (Behere et al., 2013). In many famous Hindu temples in India, such as Konark, Khajuraho, etc., naked couples are portrayed in different positions of sexual intercourse (*maithuna*) in many explicit sculptures. However, a buried secret exists behind these apparent mundane arts, and sensual positions are mostly beyond the common understanding of general spectators (Gupta, 2017). These sculptures are exhibited on the outer walls of the temple only, not inside. The inside is called the sanctum sanctorum, which is considered the soul of a temple, where the main deity is situated (Gupta, 2017). Hindu philosophy believes every human body is a sacred existence, such as a temple, and considers the existence of souls within the body as a subtle thought. "The sensuous portraits, depicting the duality of male and female energies, are only present on the outer surface of a body like the outer walls of a temple, and one needs to cross the wall-like barrier to reunite with the ultimate consciousness" (Bhattacharyya, 2020, p. 10). Hindu social culture allows intimacy and sex only in/after marriage; therefore, this relation is considered a way to cross that barrier for spouses (Bhattacharyya, 2020). Figure 12.1 illustrates the spiritual concept of marriage in Hinduism.

In ancient Hindu society, it was believed that an individual's life cycle consisted of four discrete stages ("Chatur-Ashram"), i.e., "Brahmacharya" (apprenticeship), "Garhastha" (household and family life), "Vanaprastha" (gradual retreat from family life), and "Sanyas" (renunciation). The last stage was considered an ascetic one meant for meditation and preparation for death (Chekki, 1996). In ancient Indian society, there were some orders in which individuals performed specific roles in their life course and that they were a kind of preventive measure against developing psychological problems. The Ayurveda texts described senile degeneration as "Smriti-kshaya" and "Medha-kshaya" (gradual reduction in memory and intellect) which resemble the characteristics of Alzheimer's disease and related dementia (Tiwari & Pandey, 2013). Treatment measures for dementia were also described with different herbal medicines and exercises (yoga) (Tiwari & Pandey, 2013). Physical activities in the form of yoga and meditation help prevent cognitive disorders. Although ancient Ayurvedic literature mentioned a lot of diseases along with their therapies, we still know little about them. The persons who tried to discover the journey of souls in different periods were often questioned and confused by others. However, better aging, thereby longevity, can only be achieved with positive health.

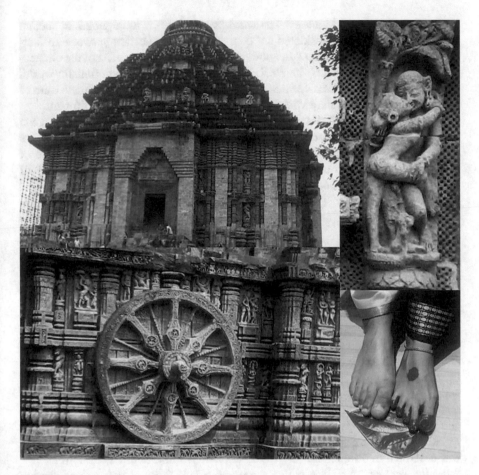

Fig. 12.1 Spiritual concept of marriage in Hinduism

12.5 The Concept of Yoga in Hinduism

Yoga, along with lifestyle modification (and self-discipline), had a profound influence on the healthy aging and well-being of ancient Indian yogis (Bhattacharyya, 2017). Therefore, before practicing yoga, one must have some basic knowledge about ancient Indian heritages. According to the census report 2011, the religion Hinduism has the largest number of followers in India (79.8% of the population) (Census of India, 2011). Unlike many other contemporary religions, Hinduism is not a well-organized religion (Nandan & Eames, 1980). Hinduism is a scientifically justified way of life. Ancient Hindu literature described different kinds of yoga practices, which individuals could adopt in their life courses, such as *Karma-yoga*, *Gyan-yoga*, *Bhakti-yoga*, *Dhyana-yoga*, *Tantra-yoga*, and *Raja-yoga*. These were not merely considered as some physical exercises but delineated as different ways (*Marg*) of life through various lifestyle modifications. These ways can uplift our souls toward the eternal journey. The word "yoga" itself is ambiguous. In ancient Sanskrit literature, it is considered as "connection," a connection between an individual and the "absolute truth." In another sense, the aim of yoga is not the connection; instead, it disconnects the *Prakriti* (the bonding of the materialistic world, which is considered the female counterpart) from the *Purusha* (the ultimate truth or "Atman," which is considered the male counterpart) to achieve that upliftment.

"Yoga-guru" Patanjali described a combination of eight different levels in yoga practice to upgrade our souls. These include "(1) 'Yama' (self-control) with five rules, i.e., non-violence, truthfulness, not stealing, chastity and the avoidance of greed; (2) 'Niyam' (observance) through purity, contentment, austerity, study of Vedas and devotion of God; (3) 'Asana' (posture); (4) 'Pranayama' (control of the breath); (5) 'Pratyahar' (restraint); (6) 'Dharana' (steadying of the mind); (7) 'Dhyana' (Meditation); and (8) 'Samadhi' (deep meditation)" (Tiwari & Pandey, 2013, p. 289).

AUM or *OM* is a sacred sound, a chanting mantra, and a spiritual icon in the Hindu religion. Its chanting produces great energy. *OM* is the origin of every sound; when expanded, it can create all the words we use in languages. The emblem *AUM* or *OM* represents three curves, a semicircle, and a dot. "A" signifies the waking state, which is represented by the large bottom curve; "U" signifies the state of dreaming, which is represented by the middle curve, whereas the upper curve "M" signifies the state of deep sleep. The dot represents the *Turiya* state, a different state of consciousness. The semicircle at the top symbolizes *Maya*, which isolates the dot from the other three curvatures. *Maya* is our affection for mundane complexities, which means that *Maya* is an illusion, an obstacle to reach the highest level of self-realization (Levine, 2011). Figure 12.2 represents the schematic diagram of the *OM* icon.

"Kundalini" is a Sanskrit word, which means "coiling up." The word *Kundalini* was described in different *Tantrik* (another ancient spiritual practice) notions as a "sleeping serpent," which is coiled three and a half times at the perineal region (*Muladhara* or the root chakra) (Hine, 1987). It was viewed as a dormant energy waiting to be awakened by specialized practices. This energy rises through the entire spinal column when unleashed, entering the chakras (psychic energy centers) one after another. When *Kundalini* rises from *Muladhara*, it crosses different chakras, i.e., *Swadhisthana* (the sacral chakra), *Manipura* (the solar plexus chakra), *Anahata* (the heart chakra), *Visuddha* (the throat chakra), and *Ajna* (the third eye chakra), one after another (Kenton, 2004). In its maximum effect, when it rises to the ultimate one, *Sahasradhara* (the crown chakra), the performer achieves "illumination" (Hine, 1987; Klostermaier, 2007). The ancient Indian yogis and sages developed this highly evolved technology through their profound devotion and worship, their research to understand how different body parts like nerves, blood, muscles, organs, and glands work together. Through breathing, posture, sound, and movement of various body parts, this technology was practiced together to achieve an ideal balance within the human body (Khalsa, 2008). The human spine consists of 33 vertebrae, of which the first 1 is the Atlas, which holds the skull (and brain/mind). According to different ancient spiritual pieces of literature, the chakras, as

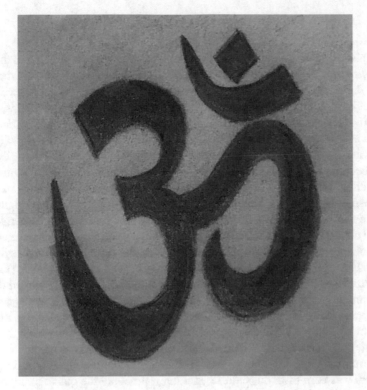

Fig. 12.2 OM icon

mentioned in the secret *Kundalini* documents as *Muladhara, Swadhisthana, Manipura, Anahata, Visuddha, Ajna, and Sahasradhara*, respectively, are located in the major vertebral junctions (e.g., thoracolumbar, lumbosacral, etc.) and resemble a close connection in their position and number to the major endocrine glands. Nerve bundles are called ganglia and are situated at the junction of different groups of vertebrae (Bentov, 1990). The rhythm of the heart muscle induces impulses to the brain, which also produces an impulse similar to that of a current loop. The *Kundalini* "rises" through a route, the spinal channel, which activates the nerve endings of the corresponding circuits. This stimulation polarizes the brain and ultimately releases a large amount of energy from the body. At that time, the body becomes a capable antenna for 7.5 Hz frequency. This frequency is similar to one of the resonant frequencies of the ionosphere. Therefore, the concerned person can pick up any information from the air (Bentov, 1990). *Kundalini* is the physiological basis of evolution, a stage in the growth of individual personality and the fountainhead of past, present, and future (Sannella, 1987).

12.6   Influence of Hinduism on Other Civilizations

Recent historical excavations revealed some surprising discoveries. One of the common myths is that Columbus discovered America, which is probably the most significant distortion of history. History proves that "when Europe was still uncivilized, Indian culture, as well as American culture, was highly advanced" (Palleres, 2005). According to ancient Indian epics, the earth was divided into seven islands (*dweepas*) after the sons of Swayambhuva Manu. America was in Krauncha *dweepam* (island). There was a forest in the Krauncha island, and its name was Kapilaranya. This forest has become what is now the state of California (Manorama, 2017). People today are searching for the way of life. The modern materialistic world is giving us apparent pleasure, but we are still desiring some unknown destination. We might get it from the spirituality of ancient India, the spirituality of the ancient Americas, the spiritual concept that was absent in the then Europe. Even Christ's messages of love were probably adulterated. His future presence on the earth as the great savior was predicted in India's "Bhavishya Purana" many years before his birth (Palleres, 2005). Ancient India can be considered a spiritual giant. It can be assumed that the Vedic literature, if thoroughly researched and understood, may emerge as a significant threat to many of our modern concepts and the current materialistic worldview.

The Indus Valley Civilization was a Bronze Age civilization and one of the oldest civilizations in the world that started flourishing around 3300 BCE, mainly in the northwestern regions of South Asia (Kulke & Rothermund, 2004). Later on, Hinduism was born from this culture, making it probably the oldest living religion in the current world. Many scholars, such as Gordon Ekholm and Chaman Lal and Ramon Mena, had compared these cultures systematically at different times. They found similarities in the cultural and social structure of Hindus and ancient civilizations of the Americas. Will Durant, an American historian, published his massive collection, *The Story of Civilizations* (comprised of 11 parts), where he mentioned Indian civilization as the most ancient (Durant & Durant, 1975). He mentioned that the then Indians explored different sea routes to reach different distant countries to spread their cultures and trades (Durant & Durant, 1975). Furthermore, even after being destroyed partially by different invaders and warriors in different periods, several pieces of ancient Indian literature on astronomy (*Jyotishya*), aeronautics (*Vimanasashtra*), medicines (*Ayurveda*), and mathematics (*Vedic Ganitsashtra*) are still considered unique and, if properly researched and understood, could uncover many legendary secrets.

The Aztec culture started in the early thirteenth century and developed in what is now Mexico and its surrounding regions. This civilization shows some striking similarities to that of the Indus Valley Civilization. In ancient American texts, it was described that a mighty warrior came from the east and married one of the Naga princesses. According to some historians, this might be *Arjuna*, the middle *Pandava*. Aztecs also divided their society into four parts, both in the domains of labor and spiritual status, as did the Hindus. There were plenty of similarities in these two cultures regarding education, marriage, death, cremation, and social life. They even worshiped nearly the same kind of idols, which are still found in museums in Central America (Palleres, 2005).

On the other hand, Mayan culture started flourishing around 2600 BC and developed in the region presently known as southern Mexico, Guatemala, and Honduras. They were renowned for their art, architecture, and mathematical and astronomical systems. It is also surprising that in all these domains, this civilization also has plenty of striking similarities with the Hindu culture of Southeast Asia, mainly India. The temples made in these two different parts of the globe have surprising similarities in architectural patterns and the rituals of worship pattern as well. The Mayans used to believe that the soul remains an integral part of the body during birth. It is only sickness or death that can separate the body from the soul, and death causes the permanent separation. Mayans believed in the afterlife (Weider, 1998). Their concept of the afterlife and reincarnation is also similar to the idea of Hinduism.

Another ancient civilization, Inca, started flourishing around the early thirteenth century in the region of present-day Peru and its surrounding areas. The Incas were famous for their art, farming, language, and the formation of governmental structures. There were similarities in nurturing astronomy in these two cultures, and the Incan sun calendar has an influence from the ancient Indian sun calendar. The Incas placed a massive emphasis on their god *Viracochas*, and Incan mythology describes that the *Viracochas* came from some distant lands beyond oceans by boat. Similarly, in Hindu mythology, a demon king (*asura*) known as *Virochana* with his few companions went out to spread divine wisdom to distant countries of the west. Finding some similarities in periods, some historians predicted that *Viracochas* (in Sanskrit, "a brave man filled with knowledge") and *Virochana* (in Sanskrit "the shining one") were the same people (Palleres, 2005).

These influences are quite significant in the discussion of souls. A 5-year-old little girl was asked by her teacher, "how many apples will you have if I give you two apples on the one hand and two apples on the other?" The girl firmly and repeatedly told her teacher that the answer would be five. The teacher was annoyed as her student was technically wrong, but the little girl was practically right as she had one apple already in her bag. It is our soul that teaches us to discover that hidden apple. It is our soul that guides us to differentiate between technical and practical rightness in every step of our life course. Therefore, without knowing the basic societal structure, the discussion of the soul becomes meaningless. The concept of the "third eye" (also called forehead dot) was symbolized among many cultures like Aztec, Mayan, and Inca, and it was originally conceptualized from Hinduism (Cassaro, 2011). As humans advanced in the process of evolution, the third eye gradually atrophied, became the modern "pineal gland," situated precisely in the geometric center of the human brain (Cassaro, 2011). This traditional third eye needs to be awakened through an ancient "Kundalini yoga" technique when the yogi (the performer of yoga) experiences "illumination" during the discovery of the soul. The Incas believed this doctrine of duality, with the *Ida* (assumed as female/the moon) and *Pingala* (assumed as male/the sun) of Kundalini yoga, and believed in a totality comprised of two opposing and contrasting forces locked in equilibrium. The

Mayans (the similar Mayan words of "yok'hah" used for "yoga" and "Kultunlilni" that refers to the divine power and is synonymous with "Kundalini") and the Aztecs also strongly believed in the same duality. How did the same idea come from two distant parts of the globe? The archaeologists have found some connections between these civilizations (Cassaro, 2011). So, there must be some common beliefs in those cultures regarding the concept of the soul's journey (even after death), influenced by Hinduism.

12.7 Conclusion

Civilizations rise and fall—history tells us that it is almost inevitable. Some rise again (like the Chinese), and some do not (like the Incas and Imperial Rome). Therefore, even for the most powerful country in the present world, it is not wise to waste resources in a casual manner. We must be aware that the natural resources we are using were present before our birth, but our next generation will suffer if we do not use them wisely. A casual and conceited feeling of greatness among the general population will inevitably lead any civilization to lose its preeminence, and significant resurgence after a fall is not always possible. Civilizations can be ended, but the journey of souls will not. We should not be asleep all the time. We have to awaken our souls to protect ourselves, our civilization, and our world. The spiritual concept of Hinduism is ideal in this way, both in life and the afterlife. At this point, it must be added that I do not claim to be a scholar of the Hindu religion. This discussion on Hinduism is neither advertising any religion nor claiming any superiority of any religion over the others. Instead, it is to convey a message that the term religion should be used as a medium or bridge to unite our thoughts with the outer world, not serve as a barrier wall that divides one human soul from another. However, the term religion has been politicized as has been the case for Hinduism, Islam, Christianity, and many others. We fail to recognize the real scenario because of this stereotyping. "Philosophy Hinduism" is much more than a mere "religion Hinduism."

If a frog lives in a well for an extended period, it cannot grow its knowledge about the outer world. We are also sitting in our small domain with the belief that the whole universe is within it. However, we need to demolish the boundary of our tiny world and enrich ourselves with the knowledge of the outer world. Also, we need to spread our knowledge to the outside to form a meaningful universe, and by that only then can we accomplish our purpose. At the same time, we should not forget our identity; blind imposition of the Western concepts on Indian thoughts (and vice versa) will only distort their significance, as the Westernization of "yoga" represents itself as mere physical exercises ("evidence-based"). Therefore, if we possess a fresh mind and holy spirit, power will come automatically within us (the Holy Bible). However, if we only make claims of being a "sage," no one will trust us. When we can acquire that power, everyone will automatically consider us as influential persons. We should always be aware that every lousy work will pull us toward a bad future, but every good work will save us from evil and take us a step ahead toward a totality. Probably the worst effect of globalization took place when the meaning of *Dharma* transformed it into its literal counterpart *religion*, and we are still carrying that meaning, ignoring our past.

References

Abhedananda, S. (1944). *Life beyond death*. Ramakrishna Vedanta Math. Retrieved from: www. spiritualbee.com/media/life-beyond-death-swami-abhedananda.pdf

Anonymous. (1968). *Brhadāranyakopanisad (sānuvāda Śānkarabhāsya sahita)*. Chapter 4, Section 4, Verse 122. Gorakhpur: Gita Press. Retrieved from: https://www.exoticindiaart. com/.../brihadaranyaka-upanishad-with-commentary-of-sh...

Anonymous. (2009). *Kathopanisat (Katha Upanishad with Four Commentaries)*. Chapter 1, Section 2, Verse 18. Gorakhpur: Gita Press. Retrieved from: www.gitapressbookshop.in/katho-panishad.html

Behere, P. B., Das, A., Yadav, R., & Behere, A. P. (2013). Religion and mental health. *Indian Journal of Psychiatry, 55*(Suppl2), S187–S194.

Bentov, I. (1990). *Kundalini*. Crystalinks. Available at: http://www.crystalinks.com/kundalini-.html

Bhattacharyya, K. K. (2017). Centenarians in India: The present scenario. *International Journal of Community Medicine and Public Health, 4*(7), 2219–2225. https://doi.org/10.18203/2394-6040.ijcmph20172809

Bhattacharyya, K. K. (2020). The sacred relationship between marriage, spirituality, and healthy aging in Hinduism. *Journal of Religion, Spirituality, & Aging, 32*(2), 135–148. https://doi.org/1 0.1080/15528030.2019.1670771

Cassaro, R. (2011). *Written in stone: Decoding the secret Masonic religion hidden in Gothic cathedrals and world architecture*. Deeper Truth Books, LLC. Retrieved from: https://www. richardcassaro.com/books-videos/written-in-stone

Census of India. (2011). *Office of the Register General and Census Commissioner, India*. Ministry of Home Affairs, Government of India. Retrieved from: http://www.censusindia.gov. in/2011census/population_enumeration.aspx

Chekki, D. (1996). Family values and family change. *The Indian Journal of Social Work, 69*, 338–348.

Das, T. K. (2019). Religion: Origin and emergence of new doctrines. *SSRN*. Retrieved from: https://doi.org/10.2139/ssrn.3330433

Durant, W., & Durant, A. (1975). 'Our Oriental Heritage.' In *The story of Civilization (Volume 1)*. MJF Books. USA. (ISBN13: 9781567310238). Retrieved from: www.akshayedges.blogspot. com/2016/01/india-mother-of-all-civilizations.html

Fontana, D. (1999). *Learn to Meditate: A Practical Guide to Self-Discovery and Fulfillment*. San Francisco, CA: Chronicle Books. ISBN 0811822508, 9780811822503.

Fowler, J. D. (2002). *Perspectives of Reality: An Introduction to the Philosophy of Hinduism*. Portland, OR: Sussex Academic Press. ISBN 1898723931, 9781898723936.

Grof, S. (2010). "The Posthumous Journey of the Soul" (ch. 5). In *The ultimate journey: Consciousness and the mystery of death* (pp. 59–95). MAPS.

Gupta, B. (2012). *An introduction to Indian philosophy: Perspectives on reality, knowledge and freedom*. Routledge.

Gupta, A. (2017). *GodSpeaksinBhagavadGita:forYoungandOld: CompleteBookofWisdomwith700 GitaVersesandEnchantingStories*. Partridge Publishing, India. ISBN 9781482888317. Retrieved from: https://www.quora.com/Why-there-are-erotic-sculptures-at-the-Sun-Temple-Konark-a...

Hine, P. (1987). *Kundalini, a personal approach*. Chaos International. Retrieved from: http://stor-age.ning.com/topology/rest/1.0/file/get/2804913459?profile=original

Srimad Bhagavad-Gita – http://www.bhagavad-gita.org/Gita/verse-02-20.html

Srimad Bhagavad-Gita – http://www.bhagavad-gita.org/Gita/verse-02-27.html
Srimad Bhagavad-Gita – http://www.bhagavad-gita.org/Gita/verse-15-08.html
Kenton, R. (2004). A kabbalistic view of the chakras. Retrieved 13 July 2021, from http://www.kabbalahsociety.org/wp/articles/a-kabbalistic-view-of-the-chakras/
Khalsa, H. K. (2008). *Physical wisdom: Kundalini yoga as taught by Yogi Bhajan*. Kundalini Research Institute. Retrieved from: https://www.amazon.com/Physical-Wisdom-Kundalini-Taught-Bhajan/dp/1934532037
Klostermaier, K. K. (2007). *A Survey of Hinduism*. State University of New York Press. ISBN 978-0791470824.
Kulke, H., & Rothermund, D. (2004). *A history of India* (4th ed., pp. 21–23). Routledge. Retrieved from: https://ipfs.io/ipfs/.../wiki/India.html
Levine, M. (2011). 5 Facts you may not know about 'OM'. *Internet Source*. Retrieved from: https://www.mindbodygreen.com/0.../5-Facts-You-May-Not-Know-About-OM.html
Lucas, S. (2014). *The seven subtle bodies of multidimensional human consciousness*. QuantumStones.com (Internet Source). Retrieved from: https://quantumstones.com/fostering-higher-vibrations-seven-subtle-bodies/
Manorama, C. (2017). *Epics of India: Where was America and other countries when Ramayana and Mahabharata was happening in India?* Retrieved from: https://surajaquarius.blogspot.com/2017/.../epics-of-india-where-was-america-and.htm...
Nandan, Y., & Eames, E. (1980). Typology and analysis of the Asian-Indian family. In P. Saran & E. Eames (Eds.), *The new ethnics: Asian Indians in the United States*. Praeger.
Ninan, M. M. (2008). *The Development of Hinduism* (pp. 17–20). Ebook. Retrieved on July 23, 2021, from: https://books.google.com/books?hl=en&lr=&id=-8RTZcjg9awC&oi=fnd&pg=PP5&dq=Thirty+three+koti+gods+in+hinduism+aditya+vasus&ots=e4AUppdRF9&sig=YTMA1WJtYrM0JTi3ZyWrokqMkxc
Palleres, R. (2005). "Who Discovered America?" *Archaeology online*. Retrieved from: www.archaeologyonline.net/artifacts/who-discovered-america
Rajhans, G. (2018). *The Gayatri Mantra*. Online source. Retrieved from: https://www.thoughtco.com/the-gayatri-mantra-1770541
Sannella, L. (1987). *The Kundalini Experience: Psychosis or Transcendence*. The Integral Publishing. Retrieved from: www.atlanteanconspiracy.com/2014/06/atlantis-and-kundalini-yoga.html
Tiwari, S. C., & Pandey, N. M. (2013). The Indian concepts of lifestyle and mental health in old age. *Indian Journal of Psychiatry, 55*(Suppl S2), 288–292.
Van Buitenen, J. A. B. (1998). Hindu sacred literature. *Encyclopedia Britannica III. Macropaedia, 8*, 923–933.
Vivekananda (undated). *The Complete Works of Swami Vivekananda* (Vol. 1). Kolkata, India: Advaita Ashrama. Retrieved from: estudantedavedanta.net/Complete%20Works%20of%-20Swami%20Vivekananda.pdf
Weider, R. (1998). *Encyclopedia of cultures and daily life* (p. 290). Detroit, MI. Retrieved from: https://wikivividly.com/wiki/Maya_death_rituals
WordZz. (2021). Are there really 33 crore gods in Hinduism? Retrieved on July 23, 2021, from: https://www.wordzz.com/really-33-crore-gods-hinduism/

Index

© The Author(s), under exclusive license to Springer Nature Switzerland AG 2021
K. K. Bhattacharyya, *Rethinking the Aging Transition*,
https://doi.org/10.1007/978-3-030-88870-1

Printed in the United States
by Baker & Taylor Publisher Services